GENDER AND SLUM CULTURE IN ASIA

GENDER AND SLUM CULTURE IN ASIA

Anil Kumar Srivastava

MD PUBLICATIONS PVT LTD
NEW DELHI
www.mdppl.com

Published by :

MD Publications Pvt Ltd
"MD House", 11, Darya Ganj,
New Delhi - 110 002
Phone : +91-11-45355555
E-mail : contact@mdppl.com
Website: www.mdppl.com

ISBN: 978-81-7533-260-7

Published and Printed by Mr. Pranav Gupta on behalf of **MD Publications Pvt Ltd** at Times Press, Delhi.

PREFACE

A slum, as defined by the United Nations agency UN-HABITAT, is a run-down area of a city characterized by substandard housing and squalor and lacking in tenure security. The term has traditionally referred to housing areas that were once relatively affluent but which deteriorated as the original dwellers moved on to newer and better parts of the city, but has come to include the vast informal settlements found in cities in the developing world. According to the United Nations, the proportion of urban dwellers living in slums decreased from 47 per cent to 37 per cent in the developing world between 1990 and 2005. However, due to rising population, the number of slum dwellers is rising. One billion people worldwide live in slums and the figure will likely grow to 2 billion by 2030.

Urbanization has led to increased productivity and economic diversification, but also deprivation, poverty, and marginalization. Environmental problems include those caused by widespread poverty and those caused by industrialization and a change in consumption patterns. The cumulative impact of these two causes has serious effects on urban dwellers, especially poor children. Low incomes, illiteracy, and inaccessibility to development opportunities further complicate problems. Slum dwellings have no ventilation or natural light and are most vulnerable. Slum dwellers suffer from dust, smoke, and noise pollution. Piles of garbage, potholes, stray animals, flies, and mosquitoes are common.

Urbanization has increased disease-producing agent, e.g., toxic chemicals and car exhaust fumes. Lead emitted from car exhausts or industry causes reduced fine motor coordination, hyperactivity, lower IQs, and perceptual problems in slum children. Few slums have access to potable water and sanitation services. Children in slums are more vulnerable to diseases and deficiencies than their rural and other urban counterparts.

Urban upgrading, poverty reduction, and pro-poor governance by increasing awareness of the link between urban violence, poverty, ineffective governance, and suitable options to mitigate urban violence and enhance public safety and security in urban areas is an immense need of today . Due to the lack of understanding of the complex nature of the problem and the link between poverty and violence has led to government policies that focus on repression and conventional policing measures, with a predictably little impact. Innovative approaches are needed to address the multifaceted nature of violence and specific security needs of the urban poor. Without this, the vision of a better quality of life for city dwellers will remain just a dream.

I am very grateful to Mr. Pranav Gupta, Director of MD Publications Pvt Ltd, New Delhi, for his kind cooperation and support for this book.

Anil Kumar Srivastava

CONTENTS

1

Urbanisation and Gender

Of the many profound changes which have swept Asia during the last half-century none have been so profound and far reaching as the doubling of the proportion of population living in urban areas. In 1950, 231 million Asians lived in urban areas and by 2000 they had increased five times to 1.22 billion while their proportions of the total population increased from 17.1 to 34.9 percent (United Nations 2001a). Moreover, in the next two decades Asia will pass the threshold of having more than half their population living in urban areas (United Nations 2002).

While there are huge variations between countries in the level of Urbanisation and later of urban growth this is indicative of substantial economic, social and demographic change in the region. The paper firstly outlines the major patterns and trends in Urbanisation and urban growth in the region. It then examines, in so far as is possible with the information available, the role of population movement in Asian Urbanisation. It then discusses a number of key issues relating to migration and Urbanisation in the region and finally a number of policy issues relating to Urbanisation in Asia are examined.

In considering urban population issues in Asia it is important to be aware of a number of difficulties associated with the conceptualization, definition and delineation of urban areas in the region. One of the most salient features of urban areas in the region is the complex and strong linkages they have with rural areas and the high degree of population mobility which occur along those linkages. This movement has blurred the distinctions between urban and rural areas with many people working in urban areas while keeping their family in and spending long periods themselves in rural areas. Moreover the definition and delineation of urban boundaries in the region not only varies greatly between Asian countries but in many is based on administrative criteria which are not effective in distinguishing urban from rural populations.

URBANISATION TRENDS

The United Nations biennial estimates of urban, rural and city populations are used here to outline the major recent and likely forthcoming trends in Asian Urbanisation and urban growth. It is important at the outset to stress what the changes have meant in terms of numbers of people since this is most indicative of the shifts in demand and need for goods and services. The massive absolute growth that has occurred in the Asian urban sector between 1950 and 2000 (from 250 million to almost 1.5 billion people), and the rural population has increased from 1.2 to 2.3 billion. On the other hand, the Asian rural population is expected to decline over the next three decades while the urban population will almost double. However, these figures mask enormous variations between individual countries and regions within Asia.

South- Central Asia is the least urbanized part of the region with less than a third (29.8 percent) of its population living in urban areas while Eastern Asia is the most urbanized (41.6 percent). By 2030 two in three residents in East Asia will live in urban areas while the urban proportion will be 44 percent in South Central Asia and 56.5 percent in Southeastern Asia. The variation is even greater between individual countries and presents United Nations estimates and projections of the number and percent of the total population of each country in urban areas. This indicates that the level of Urbanisation varies from the city-states of China-Hong Kong and Singapore to the almost totally rural countries of East Timor (7.5 percent living in urban areas) and Bhutan (7.1 percent).

It is especially important to consider trends in the largest nations. Of the 10 nations with more than 100 million residents in 2000, six were in Asia. Clearly there has been massive urban growth over the 1950-2000 period and this will at least double again except in Japan and China. Only Japan had more than a half of its population in urban areas in 2000 but by 2030 this will also be the case in China and Indonesia. It is also important to consider the tempo of change in Urbanisation and urban growth. However, it is anticipated that the rate of increase will fall to 2.22 percent per annum over the 2000-30 period and there will be an annual decline of 0.04 percent in the rural population. Hence in the current century the total net population growth in Asia will be absorbed in urban centres.

As explained in the next section this is associated with a net transfer of population from rural to urban areas and the territorial expansion of urban settlement. An important characteristic of Urbanisation in Asia has been the emergence of mega cities - large multi-nuclear urban agglomerations of more than 10 million inhabitants. No such agglomerations were in Asia in 1950 but by 1975, three of the five in the world were Asian and by 2001, 11 of the 17 global mega cities were Asian. By 2015 there will be 21 mega cities worldwide of which 12 will be in Asia, including 7 of the 10 largest. Four will be in excess of 20 million residents. However, there are substantial problems in determining mega cities. An example is the Greater Jakarta metropolitan area in Indonesia which is now one of the world's largest urban centres.

The extent of continuous urban development in Greater Jakarta compared with the official boundaries and demonstrates the extent to which Jakarta has over spilled its boundaries. In 1995, whereas 9.1 million people lived in DKI Jakarta, 15.4 million lived in the continuous built-up urban area of the metropolitan region and 20.2 million lived in all of Jabotabek which incorporates the three neighbouring Kabupaten (regencies). Between 1990 and 1995 the Jabotabek population increased by 18 percent to reach 20.2 million persons. Most of these people live and work with a strong functional connection to and incorporation in Jakarta.

It will be noted, however, that the UN estimates gave Jakarta a population of only 11.4 million in 2001. This is substantially less than the population that lived in the continuous built-up area focused on Jakarta in 1995 and these points to the problems in the UN data relating to megà cities. Hence these rates and the population sizes for several countries have to be questioned. The significance of 'megaurban' regions in the world is seen from the fact that Jones (2002, 121) has estimated that 11 percent of the total population of Southeast Asia is living in such regions.

POPULATION MOVEMENT AND URBANISATION IN ASIA

Population movement has played a key role not only in the growth of urban centres in Asia but it has strongly influenced the social, economic and demographic structure and development of those centres. From the perspective of the growth of urban centres it is apparent that net internal migration from rural areas has been substantial. While intercensal reclassification of rural areas as urban due to the lateral expansions of urban areas has been important, rural/urban immigration has been the main engine of growth. To use the example of Jakarta in Indonesia again at the 2000 census, Jakarta and the neighbouring province of West Java-Banten accounted for 8.6 million of Indonesia's 20.2 million immigrants moving into the nation's 30 provinces (42.3 percent).

United Nations (2001) estimates of the components of growth in urban areas in the 1960s, 70s and 80s and it indicate that net migration has been substantial. It is useful to focus on a single country to show the significance of population movement in Urbanisation. In Indonesia, for example, the national urban population more than quadrupled between 1961 and 1995 and the proportion living in urban areas increased from 14.8 percent to 35.9 percent. Although shifts in definition of urban areas has had some influence, growth of urban populations has been at about 5 percent per annum over the last three decades, while the rate of growth of rural populations fell from 1.63 percent per annum in the 1970s to 0.82 percent in the 1980s, to 0.16 percent in the early 1990s.

Both rural/urban migration and reclassification have played a role but both processes can be of economic and social significance since while the latter involves movement from one labour market to another, the former may reflect a change in the local labour market with the increasing availability of non-agricultural jobs seeing non-mover residents leave the agricultural sector. A substantial part of the increase in Urbanisation in Indonesia has been due to reclassification of areas from rural to urban. Gardiner and Oey-Gardiner (1991) report that the number of rural *desa* classified as urban almost doubled between 1980 and 1990 from around 3,500 to approximately 6,700. It is apparent that not only have Indonesia's urban areas recorded massive population gains during the 1980s but there also has been a huge increase in the lateral extent of urban areas.

This lateral extension of Indonesia's urban areas has tended to occur in corridors, along major transport routes radiating out from (and linking) major urban areas. In addition to the population classified as urban in the census, however, there are large numbers of rural residents, especially in Java, who work in non-agricultural occupations often based in urban or peri-urban areas by virtue of circular migration or commuting. The blurring of the distinction between urban and rural areas in Indonesia, especially Java, which was apparent in the early 1970s, has become even more apparent over the last two decades. Indeed, McGee has coined the term *kotadesasi* to describe the process whereby extensive areas in Indonesia have a complex mix of urban and rural activities.

As is the case elsewhere in Asia, the examination of rural/ urban migration in Indonesia is made difficult by the fact that:

- fIndonesian census migration data does not differentiate between urban and rural origins of migrants.

- Indonesian census data does not detect migration within provinces and a great deal of rural to urban migration occurs within provinces.

Some indication of the importance of intraprovincial rural/urban migration is evident in the results from the 1995 intercensal survey (SUPAS). Although this survey suffers from the problems associated with small clustered samples for identifying migration patterns, it gives some interesting insights into migrations within provinces. The data do not detect all interprovincial movement since it only counts movement within kabupaten and most local mobility will occur within kabupaten boundaries. There is a clear geographical separation of areas receiving net migration gains and those with net migration losses.

Net migration gains are clearly concentrated in urban areas:

- The over spilling of Jakarta's urban development into Bogor, Bekasi, Tangerang and, to a lesser extent, Serang, Karawang and Purwakarta.
- The major urban centre of Bandung over spilling into the surrounding kabupaten of Bandung.
- The regional cities of Cirebon and Sukubumi.

The predominantly rural kabupaten of the eastern and southwestern parts of the province experienced net migration losses. This pattern clearly reflects a substantial rural to urban migration pattern. In her analysis of population movement in Central Java Wahyuni (2000) found that 68.5 percent of inter-kabupaten movement was directed toward urban areas although only 31.1 percent of the non-migrant population lived in urban areas. Some 62.5 percent of interprovincial migrants moved to urban areas. Hence the movement within the province was more oriented to urban areas than that going out of the province. Moreover, that within the province involved a greater proportion of females (52.3 percent) than did the interprovincial movement (48.8 percent).

It is not just permanent migration of rural dwellers to urban areas which has influenced urban development in Asia over recent decades. There has been an exponential increase in movement between rural and urban areas involving long distance commuting or circular migration. Such mobility has a very long history in the region but it is true that modern developments in transport have facilitated an enormous expansi n in the scale, type and composition of that movement. Again, the Indonesian case is indicative. Field studies in the early 1970s demonstrated the widespread incidence and socio-economic significance of circular migration and commuting from rural to urban areas in Indonesia. While there are no substantiating data collected in censuses or national surveys it is clear that the tempo of non-permanent movement has greatly increased over the last two decades.

There are a number of case studies which demonstrate this. In particular studies which resurveyed villages studied in the early 1970s discovered a substantial increase in non-permanent moves and found that this change had been fundamental in improving the economic situation in those villages through a substantial inflow of remittances. A comprehensive longitudinal study of 37 villages in Java carried out over the period 1967-91 concluded that: Twenty five years ago many of the landless labourers on Java had very few sources of income. Now most of the landless rural families on Java have at least one person who is working outside of the village, and in a factory or service job. In all of the villages in the 1992-93 resurvey, massive migration out of the village to jobs in the larger cities and towns was recorded and only 20 percent of households depended on agriculture for their total livelihood. The bulk of the movement recorded was on a temporary basis.

The fact that those villages were deliberately selected to be representative of villages in highly accessible and low accessibility areas suggests that the scale of non-permanent rural/urban movement from Javan villages has increased exponentially in recent years and that such movement still far outweighs permanent relocation from village to city. The reasons for opting for a non-permanent migration strategy over permanent relocation include the following elements:

- This type of mobility strategy is highly compatible with work participation in the urban informal sector since the flexible time commitments allow time to circulate to the home village. Similarly, the ease of entry to the urban informal sector is a factor.
- Participation in work in both the urban and rural sectors spreads the risk by diversifying families' portfolio of income earning opportunities.
- The cost of living in urban areas (especially Jakarta) is considerably higher than in rural areas so that keeping the family in the village and 'earning in the city while spending in the village' allows earnings to go much further.
- Java's transport system is cheap, diverse and allows workers to get to their home village quickly.
- Job options in the village, especially during seasonal increases in demand for labour (such as harvesting time) are able to be kept open. Hence risk can be spread over several sources of income.
- Many informal and formal sector employers in large cities, especially Jakarta, provide barracks type accommodation for workers.
- Often the movement is part of a family labour allocation strategy in which some members are sent out of the village to contribute to the village based family's income.
- In many cases there is a social preference for living and bringing up children in the village where there are perceived to be less negative, non-traditional influences.
- Social networks are crucial in the development of this form of migration. Most temporary migrants make their initial movement with other experienced migrants or join family or friends established at the destination.
- As is the case with international migration, recruiters and middlemen of various types have played a significant role in the increasing rural to urban migration in Indonesia.

As Collier et al. (1993, 41) point out... 'Often a factory manager will meet with the head of the village to recruit young people for his factory. They sometimes would send a bus in the morning to pick up the workers'. Such a pattern of strong *mandor* (foremen), *calo* (recruiter) and *taikong* (agents) has a long history in Java and has become even more significant in recent years in encouraging migration to both formal and informal sector jobs based in urban areas. Firman (1991), for example, has demonstrated the critical role played by *mandors* in the construction industry in urban Indonesia.

While there are many similarities in the contemporary situation with respect to patterns and processes of non-permanent migration compared with the 1970s, there also have been some significant changes. Paramount among these is the increasing involvement of women in both permanent and temporary movements, especially those directed from village to city. Another change is that the increasing size of the formal sector in Indonesian cities, especially Jakarta and other large cities in Java, has led to an increasing number of migrants having to be more or less permanently settled in the city and not free to come and go to their village as frequently and readily as was possible when they worked in the informal sector.

In many cases, for example with many of the young women working in factories in and around cities like Jakarta and Surabaya, there are intentions to eventually return to settle in their village but the fixed time commitments of their work prevents them circulating to and from the village on a weekly, fortnightly or monthly basis. A final dimension of population mobility which needs to be mentioned when considering Urbanisation in Asia is international migration. Of course, international migration has not been as substantial an element in Asian Urbanisation as it has in contemporary population growth in the major cities of Euro-American societies.

Nevertheless, international migration is assuming greater significance, especially in cities in the most developed countries in the region. In Singapore, for example, it is now estimated that 19 percent of the population are foreign citizens and 27.7 percent of the workforce are foreigners. In Hong Kong, 6.7 percent of the populations are citizens of other countries. The number of foreign nationals in 2001 in Japan was 1.77 million and there were some 224,067 overstaying illegal migrants, most of them in the nation's urban areas. In cities like Kuala Lumpur and Bangkok there are also significant numbers of foreigners, although in China's and India's cities the number of foreigners in cities is quite small.

There are a number of elements in the international migration into Asia's largest cities among which the following are particularly important:

- There is an inflow of a professional and managerial group of expatriates. This group is increasing in size throughout the region and while it involves some foreigners of Asian origin, especially from India and the Philippines, skilled people from Europe, North America, Japan, Korea and Australia-New Zealand predominate. It is partly associated with increased Foreign Direct Investment in these cities and the associated transfer of staff from parent companies located in MDCs. It also includes other skilled people who are in demand because local mismatches between rapidly growing and restructuring economies demands jobs which cannot be met by the local training/ education system. All major cities in the region have significant numbers of this group but especially Singapore, Kuala Lumpur, Hong Kong and Bangkok.
- There is a substantial influx of women to work as domestic maids, especially in the cities in the Newly Developing Countries (NDCs) – Taiwan, Hong Kong, Singapore, Brunei, and Malaysia. They are predominantly drawn from Indonesia, the Philippines and Sri Lanka.
- The construction industry in many cities in NDCs is dominated by foreign workers. In several countries, too, low skilled foreign workers have been brought in to work in factories and in other low pay, low skill areas. The so-called 'entertainment', sex industry is an important element in the major cities and in several places foreigners, especially women, is involved. Undocumented workers often trafficked into the country are substantial.

- In several cities foreign workers, many of them undocumented, have become an important part of the informal sector. International migration is associated with the increasing incorporation of cities into the global economic system. It is one of the distinctive characteristics of Asia's mega cities.

The high levels of permanent and non-permanent movement to Asia's cities are important in increasing their strong linkages to their rural hinterlands, to the region and to the world. These linkages are important in shaping the social, economic and demographic characteristics of the cities but also are important conduits of money to rural areas through remittances as well as ideas and goods. Moreover, during the financial crisis of the late 1990s in several countries in the region, the chief initial impact was in urban areas and one of the ways in which urban dwellers coped with the crisis was for some family members to return temporarily to their village origins. In most cities in the region more than a half of the inhabitants are first generation migrants from rural and small urban areas or the children of those migrants. In addition, because urban origin remittances are such an important component in the economies of many rural areas in Asia, the impact of the crisis quickly spread to those areas.

ISSUES RELATING TO MIGRATION AND URBANISATION IN ASIA

URBANISATION AND ECONOMIC GROWTH

Many commentators in the past have seen cities as having a parasitic role in relation to their hinterlands; extracting their surpluses, depriving them of their most talented and entrepreneurial residents, assigning them low levels of provision of utilities and services etc. However, in Asia at least there is an emerging consensus that cities, especially the mega cities, are major 'engines of growth' in national economies. As Jones (2002, 121) has pointed out: '... Bangkok produced 37 percent of Thailand's GDP and Manila, 24 percent of the Philippines' GDP. In 1990 the ratio of city GDP per capita was

3.5 for Bangkok, 1.9 for Manila and 3.7 for Shanghai'. Over the last decade the most dynamic sectors in national economies in the region have been largely urban based activities.

Many countries in the region have deregulated and opened up their economies to outside investment and the focus of most of this investment has been the cities. Much of the foreign investment was from Japan, Taiwan, South Korea, Hong Kong and Singapore and has involved massive growth of factories to take advantage of cheap, abundant and readily controlled labour in poorer countries in the region. Industries like clothing, electrical goods, footwear, toy manufacturing which are highly labour intensive and involve much assembly type activity have been drawn to the cities of the poorer nations in the region. In recent years China has become the main focus of this investment so that the population of its largest eastern region cities is growing at unprecedented rates. However, the onset of economic crisis in several Asian countries saw a withdrawal of foreign investment from countries like Indonesia which had a substantial impact on employment in some cities.

The development of export-oriented manufacturing activity has created considerable demand for low and medium skilled labour, especially for women. It has influenced the economic structure and form of the cities with most factories being very large and located on the rapidly expanding peripheries of the cities. There have been substantial spillover effects on other parts of the urban economy, both its formal and informal sectors. Moreover, through remittances there have been impacts throughout the hinterlands of cities. While the last decade has seen rapid economic growth in large urban centres, some regional areas have suffered as a result of a concentration of power, investment, decision making and services in large cities. Contrasts between the prosperity of these cores and many peripheral areas has grown and been exacerbated by the most entrepreneurial, risk taking and educated groups from the outer regions being attracted into the centre.

The opening of national economies to outside investment has exacerbated this with most foreign investment being concentrated in the nation's largest urban areas. As a result, the largest cities have attracted a disproportionate amount of national provision of services etc. and wide gaps have grown between GDP levels per capita and growth within national spaces. In some nations, however, political changes in the late 1990s began to challenge the concentration of investment, power and resources in a few major cities. In Indonesia, for example, the fall of President Suharto in 1998 has been followed by a period of democratization and associated with this has been a major move toward devolution of decision making, revenue collection, power and investment to the regional level.

URBANISATION AND WELL-BEING

The rapid economic growth in Asia's cities in recent years has not been shared equally between all inhabitants. Indeed, there are stark inequalities evident expressed most graphically in the contrasts between opulent leafy sections of cities characterized by large housing on spacious allotments occupied by elites and the overcrowded, often unhealthy, ramshackle dwellings of the poor often located in squatter settlements on public land with little or no service provision. While the latter areas are extensive and an area of concern in Asian cities, they can often tell a misleading story to the outside observer of conditions in Asian cities. As Jones points out: 'Most indicators of welfare or human resource development, such as consumption levels, mortality rates and educational attainment, show that big city dwellers (for example, in Jakarta or Bangkok) have a considerable advantage over their rural counterparts'.

Nevertheless, within cities there are steep gradients of inequality between the haves and have nots in these cities and those differences may be increasing. In most countries in the region infant mortality levels are generally lower in urban areas than in rural, especially in the largest cities. Formal poverty measures usually indicate that poverty levels are lower in urban areas, although there are real difficulties in equating costs of living in urban and rural areas in Asian contexts. Nevertheless, there are large populations living below the poverty lone, however different, in Asian cities. Moreover, family based support systems may be weaker in urban areas than they are in rural areas for many groups.

THE INFORMAL SECTOR

One of the most distinctive features of the economies in most Asian cities is the fact that in most, more than half of workers are employed in the urban informal sector. These are jobs which generally do not have fixed hours, are in family rather than formal enterprises, are small scale, often lack a fixed location, involve small investments, have no fixed earnings, involve no formal training, lack formal security and are not within the formal economy in terms of regulations, work conditions, taxation etc. They involve provision of a myriad of services at the individual or household level, small scale selling and a wide range of skilled and semi-skilled trades. They often provide services to households but also are involved in a wide array of manufacturing and service activities and often are linked in complex ways with the formal sector.

A major characteristic is that it is highly absorptive with new workers being able to readily enter it, largely through family, friendship or locality of origin connections than through possessing formal qualifications. Accordingly, new entrants to the city often enter the labour market through the informal sector. Moreover, the informal sector's flexible hours and work week regime make it highly compatible with circular migration. Working in the formal sector usually involves set daily hours and working weeks which mean that its workers need either to settle in the city or commute in daily from the environs in the city. Indeed, very long distance commuting has become characteristic of Asia's largest cities involving an array of transport types but especially buses and railways. Very often, there is strong occupational segmentation in particular areas of the informal sector so that urban workers in particular occupations tend to come from the same areas of origin.

While the bulk of informal sector activity is relatively small scale, particular activities can grow to be quite large. Some informal sector activity takes place on the margins of law and indeed there are some activities which are considered illegal by city authorities. Interpretations of the role of the informal sector in Asia's cities have changed over recent decades. An early view saw the sector as being more of a 'sink' to absorb the surplus of workers in such cities and an area for migrants to work until they got a 'real job' in the formal sector. This view has changed with there being increased recognition of the important role that the sector plays in the economy of Asian cities and economies.

WOMEN, MIGRATION AND URBANISATION

One of the distinctive features of rural to urban migration in Asia has been the importance of women in that movement, a feature which has differentiated it from other parts of the world. Patterns vary from country to country but in many Asian countries historical and cultural factors have combined with particular developments in the industrial and service sectors of cities to expand employment opportunities for women. A United Nations study has found from examination of sex ratios of rural-urban migration flows in several countries, that it is in Asian countries that the greatest feminization of flows have occurred. Among the Asian countries studied, there were 116.8 males to every 100 female rural-urban migrants in the 1960s but this declined to 111 in the 1970s and 96.6 in the 1980s.

There are variations between countries but generally there has been an increase in the involvement of women in rural-urban migration throughout the region due to:

- Increased growth of export based large scale manufacturing and assembly activities in Asian cities. For many of the activities in those new factories (assembly of electric devices, clothing, shoe manufacture, toy manufacture etc.)

women are preferred by employers because they are generally paid lower wages, are considered more easily controlled and are considered better able to undertake tasks which involve delicate and intricate finger work as well as repetitive tasks. The bulk of these women has high school level education and is directly recruited from rural areas and lives in dormitories or shared accommodation. Employers often exploit these women and there is a tendency to dismiss them once they get into the family formation age group, so there is a high turnover.

- As the cities have expanded, there has been a rapid increase in demand for domestic workers as both the middle and upper classes conventionally employ several domestics. The great majorities are women and they are almost all recruited from rural areas.
- There is also evidence of more women moving independently for educational and employment reasons to cities. In recent decades, traditional sanctions on the independent movement of women have been eroded with increased education and the breakdown of strong patriarchal, extended families.
- The informal sector of cities has many opportunities for females, especially in small scale selling and service activities. Both permanent and circular migrants are involved in this area.
- There has been substantial growth of the sex and entertainment industries of Asian cities and women involved in these are almost entirely rural-urban migrants and circulators.

A key characteristic of Asian cities has been that their female labour forces tend to be much more occupationally segregated than is the case for their male counterparts. In some of these areas of work there are opportunities for exploitation, not only in work that occurs in homes (domestics), and in illegal or quasi legal contexts (sex work) but also in more formal work situations like in factories. However, it is clear that social networks offer some protection in these situations.

Increasing levels of female workforce participation outside the home are characteristic of Asian cities throughout the region.

There is strong evidence of marriage ages being considerably higher in cities than in rural areas and fertility levels being considerably lower. Indeed, several Asian cities have fertility levels below replacement level (e.g. Jakarta, Bangkok) and indeed some (e.g. Shanghai) have some of the lowest contemporary fertility levels in the world.

PLANNING AND ENVIRONMENTAL ISSUES

The rapidly growing and large populations of Asian cities presents before the city planners with an array of daunting challenges in provision of appropriate services, utilities and infrastructure. Indeed, the sheer size of multinuclear mega cities is especially difficult in this aspect. An important issue relates to governance. In fact, many of the largest urban areas have administrative and planning boundaries which have little relationship to functioning cities. Hence, integrated planning can be very difficult with a number of jurisdictions having responsibility for different parts of the city and policies often being at odds with one another. City administrators often lack the power and organisation to apply an appropriate and equitable taxation and revenue raising system and to fully enforce building codes, environmental controls etc. Many cities in the region hence face environmental problems of substantial magnitude.

In Jakarta in Indonesia, air pollution levels in some parts of the city often exceed WHO maximum levels, a situation exacerbated by the universal use of leaded petrol. Availability of uncontaminated fresh water is an issue in many areas. In Jakarta overuse and contamination of aquifers is a large problem and incursion of sea water into those aquifers is making it impossible to draw fresh water from wells over a large part of the city. An array of health problems associated with exposure to emissions, infected water etc. are serious. Congestion has reached massive proportions in several cities, although some have developed modern rapid transit systems.

Public transport is the main way people get around in the cities and while there is a diverse range of such transport available, travel times within cities are much greater than in European and North American cities of comparable size.

Other utilities such as electricity are difficult to provide on a reliable and economic basis. Sewerage is confined to limited parts of most cities and waste disposal is a massive problem. Some cities have substantial problems in maintenance of law and order and crime is a major issue. Cities are unable to meet the challenge of providing adequate or indeed in some case any housing to the burgeoning urban populations. Squatter settlements have hence developed in railway right of way areas and in other public land areas. Provision of health, education, policing, aged care and other services is difficult.

THE AGE STRUCTURE OF ASIAN CITIES

One of the most consistent of findings in relation to rural-urban migration all over the world is the age selectivity of that movement. This is evident which shows the median age specific rates of rural out migration of a sample of countries in three major world regions over the 1960s, 1970s and 1980s. This shows the concentration in the young adult age groups and these points to Asian cities having considerably younger age structures than rural areas.

A number of things follow from this, such as the increasing problem in some rural areas where aged parents are not able to receive assistance in old age from children as much as used to be the case because the children have moved to the city. In the city, however, there are large concentrations of young adults placing considerable pressure on education services but also on the labour market to continue to be able to absorb each year large numbers of people entering the labour market for the first time.

This concentration of the young also tends to be selective in that it tends to be the more highly educated youth population which moves to the city and these tend to have relatively high levels of unemployment. In Asian cities, unemployment levels are low by European standards because the poor cannot afford to be unemployed where there is no formal social security system. Accordingly, they have to take on any work regardless of its status, remuneration etc. Hence unemployment in such contexts tends to be concentrated in the more educated groups whose family can afford to support them until they are able to get work commensurate with their aspirations and level of qualifications.

Hence Asian cities have disproportionate concentrations of young, better educated people. In some rural Asian urban contexts they also have very high levels of unemployment. Some have argued that this can lead to the development of a large disaffected group who feel disenfranchised and not able to get good jobs in manifestly expanding areas of the economy. When this is allied to a perception of corruption and nepotism at high levels it can lead to discontent, protest and opposition to the status quo. Hence the conflicts against authority in some Asian countries tend to be started by young urban based people.

MIGRATION, URBANISATION AND HEALTH IN ASIA

There are a number of health implications which flow from developments in Urbanisation and population mobility in Asia. The movements of people from different ecological contexts means migrants may not have antibodies to cope with new localized diseases. Many newcomers to urban areas in Asia live in cramped unhealthy situations. Some workers may sleep outdoors or be exposed to infectious diseases through contaminated food and water. This may be partly due to migrants, especially circular migrants, wishing to maximize the amount of earnings that they are able to remit to their home areas.

One area which is of increasing concern is HIV/AIDS. While in most countries in Asia prevalence levels are relatively low, there are some indications that it could spread quite rapidly and that one of the main vehicles for this is the high levels of population mobility, especially that between rural and urban areas. There is growing recognition of an important nexus between labour mobility, the expanding commercial sex industry and HIV infection in Asia.

As indicated earlier, the commercial sex industry has grown rapidly in Asia and its main location is in urban areas. Moreover, the sex industry often locates in areas within cities where there are large numbers of migrant workers who are a group who are major users of the commercial sex sector. This is because most migrant workers, especially the circular migrants, are young males who are freed from the close sanctions on their activity in the home area, if married they are separated from wives and family, they often have cash available and are lonely and separated from other life in the city.

Hence the opportunities for contracting HIV infection are considerable, especially in the situation in Asia where the use of condoms for commercial sex is not well established. In several countries high rates of infection have been found among sex workers and some groups of mobile workers. The infected workers then return to their home areas and to other urban work destinations and have potential to spread the disease. Moreover, most sex workers are migrant workers themselves and can contract the disease and spread it to their home village and to other urban areas since most do not work in a single city.

POLICIES REGARDING URBANISATION

Several countries in Asia have adopted policies and programmes which attempt to intervene in the processes of Urbanisation and labour mobility. For much of the period of the 1970s and 1980s strong anti-urban sentiments prevailed in some governments and international agencies. This saw rapid urban growth as having deleterious effects, both in urban areas through excessive demands being placed on utilities, housing, transport, waste collection, job opportunities, health and education services etc. as well as rural areas being robbed of their most talented and entrepreneurial people which was a barrier to economic and social development in those areas.

This led to a rash of anti-urban policies and programmes such as:

- In some cases cities were 'closed' so that people who were not registered residents and who were detected at check points were evicted from the city. This, for example, was the case for Jakarta in the early 1970s.
- In several large Asian cities squatter settlements, whose inhabitants were frequently migrant workers, were bulldozed.
- In some cities economic activity favoured by migrant workers was made illegal. This includes street vendors and street based service providers.

The informal sector in large cities absorbed the bulk of unskilled incoming migrant workers and programmes sought to close down many such activities. These anti-urban approaches were also influenced by somewhat romanticized notions of the 'rural way of life' being intrinsically better than in urban areas. There were elitist views that the 'privileges' of living in the city should not be open to any citizen who wishes to live there. Foreign observers were strongly influenced by contrasts of the superficial, rustic, attractive greenness of villages to the squalor of urban squatter settlements but ignored the fact that people could get work in the city but not in their village.

The fact was that anti-urban policies seemed to fly in the face of market forces:

- There was considerable 'urban bias' in both public and private investment which meant that new job creation was strongly concentrated in sectors (manufacturing and services) which were mainly urban based. On the other hand, in the agricultural sector increased commercialization, mechanization and replacement of labour inputs with capital inputs was displacing labour.
- In some cases there were other policy interventions which greatly favoured urban areas. In Indonesia, for example, the government fixed the price of the staple food, rice,

for admirable welfare reasons. However, what this meant was the urban dwellers were able to purchase their basic food at below market prices and farmers were compelled to sell their main product for less than what it was worth. Hence there was a strong advantage in favour of urban living and a disadvantage to remaining in agriculture.

- There were widening differentials between rural and urban areas in service provision in health, education etc. as well as in the availability of electricity and other utilities.
- Migrant workers in cities were showing a great deal of ingenuity and self-reliance and were not heavily dependent on governments and institutions but more on social networks based on family or origin linkages.

Hence for the bulk of immigrants they obtained their work and housing not through government and formal institutions but through family based and self-help activity in the informal sector and squatter housing. The migrants were succeeding in the city to obtain work and housing with little or no assistance from the formal institutions in the city. A critique of the anti-urban position developed through the 1980s and 1990s which was based upon several elements including:

- The realization that there were strong economic gradients between rural and urban areas and that any attempt to dissuade people from moving along them would be difficult and destine to failure.
- There was a growing body of research that indicated that the informal sector was not simply a sink which absorbed surplus labour but that it was a major productive element in the urban economy. Moreover, it had important labour absorptive capabilities that greatly facilitated people being able to enter the labour market. It was also recognized that there was considerable upward mobility in the sector.
- Similarly, research began to show that with such rapid population growth it was simply not possible for the formal constructive sector to provide sufficient housing that conformed to formal restrictions and regulations which would accommodate the growth. 'Self-help'

squatter housing often succeeded where the formal construction sector failed. Latin American work suggested that it was better to adopt a 'site and service' approach where minimal services are supplied to squatter areas.

- Another body of research showed that in Asia it is not appropriate to have separate 'urban' and 'rural' policies and programmes since there are strong and developing rural/urban ties.

Theres are flows of people, information, finance and goods along these linkages which mean that policies instituted at one end will have impacts on the other. There hence is a need when considering intervention to take into account effects in both urban and rural areas. In most countries this has led to an abandonment of anti-urban policies, although there are remnants. Indeed, Jakarta's 'closed city' legislation abandoned in the mid 1970s was revived by the Governor of Jakarta in 2001. Currently, however, a number of other elements are important:

- Firstly, in recognition of the fact that there are increasing pressures on many urban areas and lagging in many rural areas, there is increased emphasis on integrated regional, rather than urban, development strategies which self-consciously attempt to reduce the rural/urban economic gradient along which migration occurs. This emphasizes decentralisation of government activity, investment and decision making to encourage the growth of employment opportunities in regions. In addition, there is an effort to reduce the differential in service provision in such areas as health, education and electricity. It is often associated with development of devolution and democratization policies.
- Secondly, within urban areas there is less emphasis on policing and placing barriers in the way of migrants being integrated into urban labour and housing markets.

Instead, there is more of an 'accommodationist' approach which accepts:

a. Migration to the city will continue,

b. There are insufficient resources to fully provide for them.

This approach tends to facilitate their integration into the city and build on the self-help and network based support that already exists. Hence site and service schemes, upgrading of squatter settlements etc. can improve the accommodation available. Productivity in the informal sector can be enhanced by access to loans, training etc. While this brief account has overly simplified and generalized a diverse range of approaches to Urbanisation in Asia over the last four decades, it is no doubt true to say that there has been a general move away from policies and programmes which seek to act in the opposite direction to market forces and to facilitate positive trends. In the process there has been a move away from a concept of Urbanisation as somehow being unnatural and parasitic toward it being inevitable and integral in improving economic and social wellbeing.

Urban areas will soon house more than a half of Asia's population while two generations previously, only one in ten Asians lived in urban areas. This represents a profound change in the way in which Asians live their lives. However, there are many challenges which Asian Urbanisation presents to policy makers, planners and researchers. One crucial area lies in the arena of data collection and research. Planning for efficiency and equity in Asian cities requires timely and relevant research.

However, in Asia, as elsewhere, conceptualization and definition of urban areas has remained mired in the thinking of the 1970s and does not capture the nature of contemporary dynamic urban systems. Moreover, data collection systems are based on large areas while modern technology allows small building block units for censuses and other data collection which in turn allows flexible and appropriate definition of urban boundaries. Sound planning and governance of urban centres in Asia requires better delineation of boundaries and of appropriate specifically disaggregated data within those boundaries. Moreover, research in urban areas needs to be integrated so that an understanding of the dynamics of population change in urban areas may be achieved.

2

Migration and Gender

Large-scale movements of voluntary and forced migrants have uprooted more than 150 million people worldwide. Correspondingly, there has been an increased amount of attention given in both scholarship as well as pedagogy to the complexities of these movements of people, caused by varied reasons ranging from economic opportunity, ethnic violence, to social and political persecution. Economic globalization and the end of the cold war have led to the steady rise in cross-border flows since 1990, when there were an estimated 120 million migrants. According to a report by the International organisation of Migration (IOM), "As of the year 2000, there are an estimated 150 million international migrants...the 21st century is likely to continue to see large scale movements of people, both voluntary and forced."

The top 10 receiving countries - the United States, India, Pakistan, France, Germany, Canada, Saudi Arabia, Australia, the United Kingdom and Iran-accounted for 55 percent of all international migrants in 1990, and continue to host large immigrant populations. The impact of this movement on the transformation of processes of creating cultural and ethnic community, the invention of Diasporas and imagined nations, necessitates going beyond the focus on the borders and boundaries of nation-states which contain migrants, to examine the links amongst different "areas" or "regions" which send and receive flows of people. Rather than focusing on particular nation-states, recent scholarship such as by Arjun

Appadurai and Saskia Sassen has begun to examine this transnational movement of people in more global contexts.

ON SOUTH ASIAN MIGRATION

In the light of the resurgence of a transnationally linked communal violence since the 1960s in India, and the international rise of ethnic conflict in both Western and decolonized nations in the twentieth century, an urgent issue that demands scholarly attention is ethnic violence, and how it effects particular temporary and permanent migration and displacement of both individuals as well as communities, in its articulation with discourses of national as well as cultural unity, purity, and collectivities. The case of South Asia is pertinent here: the largest migration of South Asians occurred in 1947, accompanying the partition of the sub-continent into two nations India and Pakistan on the basis on religion -on the basis of religious differences and anxieties about minoritization after independence.

In the nine months between August 1947 and the spring of the following year, by unofficial counts, at least 18 million people -Hindus, Sikhs and Muslims - were forced to flee their homes and became refugees; at least a million were killed in communal violence. The scale and nature of violence that India's partition involved makes it one of the most violent events in the history of nation- formation. In the nine months between August 1947 and the spring of the following year, by unofficial counts, at least 18 million people - Hindus, Sikhs, and Muslims - were forced to flee their homes and became refugees; at least a million of them were killed in communal violence.

Yet, until the last decade or so, this mass migration - its social, political and cultural impact - has received little attention. This migration has been approached largely in the mode of documentary historical scholarship which has tended to focus on two themes:

a. The politics of Partition and the formation of the nation-state whose protagonists are the male, nationalist elite - namely, Nehru, Gandhi, Jinnah, and Mountbatten most often;

b. The regional impact of this violence and displacement in the partitioned states of Punjab and Bengal.

More recently, revisionist historiography and anthropology, as well as state governments, have begun to examine the experience of refugees and migrants, focusing particularly on the experiences of ordinary people, women and children, who were witness to violence and who became refugees of Partition. Recently, several historians and cultural critics have analyzed how the Indian nation is represented in popular literature, drama, and other public media, to reveal the gendered forms of nationalist identity in colonial and newly independent India. Pioneering work in anthropology and feminist historiography by Veena Das, Urvashi Butalia, Ritu Menon and Kamala Bhasin, has investigated women's and refugee experiences of the violence in 1947; they have also attempted to map out the complex forms of agency at work in women's negotiation of memory, nationality, and state ideology and functioning in its aftermath.

However, these studies' focus on contemporary interviews and individual testimony as the primary form of evidence, need to be supplemented by studies of middle-class cultural production in the public sphere that negotiated this experience of displacement, in order to understand how these new cultural geographies enable us to rethink nationalism, and understand the public developments and discourses that shape the testimonies and memories of those interviewed. Recent studies of nationalism foreground how print media - novels, journals and newspapers - become key technical means for representing the nation, and so for constituting national consciousness. By institutionalizing a common language, and creating a public sphere that mediates between the state and civil society, these media generate mass reading publics that form a collective imagined community - the nation.

In addition to literature and journalism, film technology emerges as a powerful and popular means of representing the nation and its populations. Hence, mass media in the public sphere are key sites to examine and address the complexities and conflicts of migration, refugee status, and human rights. However, this mass migration, and its cultural impact still needs to be examined in a transnational context, without its centering within the boundaries of the nation-state, be it India or Pakistan. Further, the construction of categories and communities like 'refugees' and 'nation' needs to be reconceived in a less regional and more transnational context - in relation to both, the history of post-Independence India, and the largely post-1950 history of global migration.

Just as many Partition refugees eventually migrated to the USA or UK in the fifties and sixties, much of the recent writing on Partition and its effects has emerged from diasporic South Asian intellectuals who have migrated to the West. In an international context, this has led to renewed attention to the problem of ethnic violence and its attendant effect of internal displacement. In this, the particular study of the gendered nature of migration has begun to receive serious attention only in the last decade or so. The different experiences of female migrants, the different conditions under which they migrate, and their differential reception in the countries they migrate to have also now garnered increased attention. A significant new trend is the increasing number of female migrants, but these women are especially vulnerable to hardship, discrimination, and abuse.

Women now make up 47.5 percent of all international migrants, and many females relocate abroad as principal wage earners rather than as accompanying family members. "They have limited access to employment and generally earn less than men and than native born women. Legally, many migrant women are vulnerable if their residence is dependent upon a relationship with a citizen or a 'primary immigrant,'" according to the IOM report. Further, in the study of migration, it is important to examine both the specificity of those migrants who are refugees, and their cultural and political reception, experience, and impact. Recent work on refugees and human rights like Jacqueline Bhabha and Liisa Malkki has begun this important work to understand the social processes by which migrants become refugees, and refugees' experiences in forging new relations of Diaspora, assimilation and cultural and national belonging.

In addition, this elides the problem of internal displacement, within nation-states, that comprises a significant part of the world's migration, yet receives less attention given its confinement within a particular nation-state's borders. Since the end of the Cold War, increasing numbers of people have been forced to leave their homes as a result of armed conflict, internal strife, and systematic violations of human rights. Whereas refugees crossing national borders benefit from an established system of international protection and assistance, those who are displaced internally suffer from an absence of legal or institutional bases for their protection and assistance from the international community.

Recent scholarship like Roberta Cohen and Francis Mading Deng's Masses in Flight: The Global Crisis of Internal Displacement analyzes the causes and consequences of displacement, including its devastating impact both within and beyond the borders of affected countries. It sets forth strategies for preventing displacement, a special legal framework tailored to the needs of the displaced, more effective institutional arrangements at the national, regional, and international levels, and increased capacities to address the protection, human rights, and reintegration and development needs of the displaced. Finally, mass human trafficking has emerged as a trend in China, while smuggling networks have been uncovered in Europe, including Germany, Hungary, Italy, Spain and the Czech Republic.

According to this report, "Many trafficked migrants find themselves forced into prostitution and/or effective slavery to pay off their debt to the traffickers or otherwise dependent on jobs where they suffer severe exploitation and abominable working conditions." The United States is by far the largest recipient of international migrants, with about 25 million foreign-born residents at the end of the 1990s. At the same time, this does not include the populations of illegal immigrants which is harder to account for: unauthorized migrants in Europe - including ethnic Albanians from Kosovo, Kurds from Iraq and Roma (gypsies) from eastern Europe - were estimated at three million in 1998, up from about two million in 1991.

This figure does not include illegal migrants in the rest of the world, and points to the centrality of ethnic conflict as a leading cause of displacement and migration. Hence, attention to international migration must needs attend to the problem of ethnic conflict and violence in a transnational perspective, as well as to the political economy of globalization, in conjunction with an examination of the cultural production of locations of community that transcend national borders, as many scholars have begun the work of. Migration has long been a topic of historical and sociological inquiry, particularly in the United States, a nation built by immigrants, and in its most utopian formulation, conceived as a refuge for them.

Theories dealing with the immigrant experience emerged in the early twentieth century in the wake of the massive wave of "new immigration" from Southern and Eastern Europe. The Chicago School of Sociology formulated many of these, by far the most powerful and the one which would generate intense historical debate was assimilation: the notion that immigrants would over time lose their "old world" traits and allegiances and become "American." While the pace of assimilation, as well as the nature of the society into which immigrants integrated was construed differently, the basic premise that immigrants moved along a trajectory towards greater homogeneity with an Anglo-American core endured for decades.

In this way, assimilation was fundamentally a teleological model under girded by the modernization principle: peasants left rural environments and immigrated to the American city where they adopted new social values - individualistic, rational and competitive. As Jon Gjerde notes, much of the early scholarship favored botanical metaphors to describe this process. Immigrants were, for example, "transplanted" or "uprooted," while the city was a "jungle" constantly invaded and reorganized by new waves of immigrants. Culinary metaphors also abounded, perhaps the most enduring of these was popularized by a Jewish immigrant, Israel Zwangill, and in his 1908 play entitled *The Melting Pot.*

SALIENT SHIFTS IN THE LITERATURE

In the 1960s, the assimilation paradigm received its first major systematic reformulation. Sociologist Milton Gordon distinguished between "cultural assimilation," and the adoption of the cultural norms of the Anglo-Saxon center, and "structural assimilation," that is, entrance into its primary institutions, including clubs and cliques. He argued that the first pattern had prevailed over the second, since ethnic groups had retained their own organizational networks. Nathan Glazer and Daniel Patrick Moynihan, intrigued by the persistence of ethnic group solidarity in New York, went further and declared that assimilation hadn't happened.

It was historians, in particular, who undermined the central arguments of the assimilation thesis by focusing on the meaning and content of ethnicity in American life. The idea, for example, that the immigrant experience was one of alienation, and that immigrants had in Oscar Handlin's famous thesis, been "uprooted" from their traditional folk ways and wrenched into the disorientating pace of modern American life was challenged by a new wave of scholarship that focused on the continued vitality and adaptability of immigrant culture. Rudolph Vecoli, for example, showed how the very idea of a static "old world" culture was problematic, and that preexisting institutions and senses of identity, rather than be a hindrance to immigrant adaptation in the United States, facilitated the process.

The focus on immigrant agency and on the dynamic networks that sustained migration flows helped refines the study of population movements as a whole. The classic "push-pull" model could simply not stand in the face of the complex phenomena with which scholars were faced, and patterns like "chain," "circular" and "career" migration could better describe the varying motivations, destinations, and timing of migrations. The move away from the assimilation paradigm towards ethnicity was linked to broader cultural and political developments, especially the Civil Rights movement, feminism, and identity politics. Coupled with the techniques of the new social history, the shift to ethnicity produced a fascinating range of material on individual ethnic groups, particularly of South European origin.

The intensive focus on one particular group, however, usually studied in one locale, tended to isolate groups from each other, and to avoid larger processes of integration. While the concept of assimilation was seriously challenged, it has not altogether disappeared. Indeed, as Russel Kazal argues, three of the most interesting areas of immigration scholarship have "revisited assimilation." Labor historians, for example, have looked at how labor activism and industrial unionism created a more unified working class out of diverse ethnic and racial base. This process of "trans-ethnic homogenization" has been tackled in a different way by scholars like David Roediger and Noel Iganatiev who place "whiteness" and its attendant privileges, at the center of their inquiry.

In doing so, they have opened up a field which had not adequately addressed questions of racial identity in the assimilation process. The fact remains that "white" ethnics have more readily assimilated into the category American than have people of color. As Roediger remarks, "becoming white and becoming 'American' were intertwined at every turn." Finally, a third group of scholars have focused on how the invention of ethnicity is part of a larger process of cultural and structural adaptation in which groups shape a pluralistic America. Immigrants do not in other words fit into an already-constituted American pattern but interact with local cultures. This interaction produces a new synthesis which shapes the wider national culture.

Besides reconceptualizing assimilation, historians have developed more sophisticated understandings of movement across space and time. The concept of transnationalism, for example, has become increasingly popular as a way to theorize modern migration. In its simplest definition transnationalism connotes back and forth movement and the creation of networks across borders, which is in fact a very old characteristic of migration. Thus, the "trade diasporas" like the Genoese in the Spanish Habsburg Empire could be viewed as a precursor to transnationalism, as could the circular labor migrations of 19th and first half of the 20th centuries, the best example in the United States context being the migration of Mexicans into the American Southwest.

However, what is new about modern migrations, and which makes a more complex understanding of transnationalism appropriate, is their connection to a whole set of cultural, economic and political exchanges that transcend the nation-state. Most importantly, these exchanges are facilitated and made more rapid by the use of technology in transportation and communications: the fax, the internet, the direct flight, the mobile phone, what Portes et al. call "space-and-time compressing technology." To a certain extent, new transnational perspectives are picking up on themes found in earlier historical and sociological work which insisted on the importance of the pre-migratory context in shaping patterns of transatlantic migration.

The work of Bernard Bailyn and Leslie Page Moch, for example, revealed the high level of internal European migration that preceded overseas migration. Saskia Sassen also focused on internal and international migration and documented its relationship to global capital. Indeed, Sassen and others have challenged what was once a basic premise of capitalist expansion, namely that labor stays local, and capital moves globally. Transnational perspectives in immigration history have thus benefited from earlier historical and sociological work that pushed open the geographic boundaries of migration studies. As a result, historians have increasingly shifted away from the rigid dichotomy between "homeland" and "host-country" and on the excessive focus on how immigrants became "American."

The contributions of anthropology have gone furthest in developing a theory of transnationalism that focuses not just on exchanges, or the rapid movement of people and information across national boundaries, but on a diasporic public sphere. While migrants are the most logical participants in this sphere, it is not exclusively their creation for what is central to the maintenance of modern transnational bonds is shared imagination. In this way, lesbians and gays have created queer transnational communities, just as a growing American Muslim community has become linked to a wider Muslim Diaspora thanks to the internet.

Transnationalism can help historians discover links that they did not previously see and to rethink the boundaries of area studies. Modern Middle East history, for example, dominated as it is by a historiography of the nation and of nationalism, might look very different if it incorporated Lebanese, Syrian and other Diasporas into its central problematic: how do people imagine them as belonging to a nation?

Surely it is not mere coincidence that the earliest proponents of Arab nationalism were Syrian, many of them emigrants themselves, and that their emphasis on culture, language, shared experience, political rights, and not on a particular piece of the map, made eminent sense to a Syrian "nation" where as many as one in six persons lived and worked in the Americas. To be sure, there are methodological problems, particularly for historians who view place as the principal generator of documents (birth certificates, marriage records, etc.), but transnational frameworks will require collaborative effort and they will generate a scholarship that more accurately reflects the complexity of the immigrant experience and imagination.

Temporary labour migration now affects most countries of the world and displays several major trends. One of the important trends is that a large number of women participate in the global labour market as principal migrant. Even though a large group of women migrated in the past, they did so as part of family migration. Moreover, causes and effects of their migration were assumed to be similar to that of men's. Over the years, several researchers contributed to the literature on the diverse experiences of woman migrants as short term contract workers, permanent residents or migrants through marriage.

Migration is a complex process. There are diversities as well as commonalities with respect of challenges that migrants of different countries of origin face. This chapter concentrates on the participation of women of Asia in the short term international labour market. It highlights the diverse experiences of migration of women from various Asian countries, and tries to link this diversity to migration policies of their countries of origin and gender determined demands for labour in the destination countries.

Over the last 25 years, the number of international migrants has almost doubled. In the 1980, 99 million people were living outside their country of origin. In 2005 it became 190 million (UN 2007). Compared to the 1960s, growth rate of migrant populations is rather high.

This is perceived by some quarters, particularly those representing the receiving countries as a concern. Nonetheless as a proportion of world's total population it remains rather modest. Women constituted just under half (49.6%) of all international migrants in 2005 (UN 2007). Significant share of women in international migration has been noted since 1960s. According to region wise estimated numbers, Asia stands as the second largest. In 2005 the total number of Asian migrants was 53 million, only surpassed by Europe which had 64 million. Asia is the second largest region with regard to total stock of migrants. The proportion of women migrants in Asia compared to other regions is the lowest in the world.

Female migration from Europe constitutes the highest percentage (53.4%) with Oceania 51.3%, North America 50.4%, Latin America and Caribbean 50.3% and Africa 47.4%. In other words, except Asia and Africa the number of women migrants exceeded the number of male migrants. Nonetheless, over the last decade's growth rate of female migrants compared to male, is higher in Asia. Since the 1980s Asian women constituted the majority of migrant workers in countries such as the Philippines, Indonesia and Sri Lanka. A large number of female migrants in Asia go through irregular channels. So, they are not recorded in the official figures.

FOUR MAJOR TYPES OF MIGRATION

Asia has been in the forefront of migration of people all along. People of Asia moved across territory for better life and livelihood. Colonial rule added new dimensions in migration. After the abolition of slavery colonial masters engineered indentured labour and moved people from Asia to all over the world. Since the 1950s many Asian countries experienced international movements mostly of professional and students to Europe, North America, Australia and New Zealand. Over the years Asia has been experiencing increased movements within the region. This has been marked by the growth of temporary short term contract migration. This has created a major scope for movement of semi- and low skilled workers along with professionals and skilled workers.

Another important trend in migration within Asia is the emergence of women as principal migrants. In case of migration of women four broad streams are discernable:

a. Typical migration of women as dependent spouses of male migrants both within and beyond Asia;
b. Independent migration of women for labour;
c. Independent migration of women as students and professionals and
d. International marriage migration.

Since the 1950s a large section of Asian males went to the developed world to study and subsequently took up employment. Another group of male migrants of Asia went to developed countries as labour migrants. Under the family reunification policy of the receiving countries these male migrants sponsored their spouses to the countries of their residence. Labour migration within Asia in its current form mostly started in the 1970s. The price hike in oil in the Gulf created scope for major infrastructural development in these countries.

This resulted in large scale migration of all categories of workers - professionals, skilled, semi skilled and low skilled. With a few exceptions all these migrants were men. The Gulf States took these workers to perform tasks under specific contracts and once the contracts were over the migrants were meant to leave. Except for the professionals and the highly skilled other migrants were not permitted to bring their spouses. This is why although 30 to 35 percent of the combined population of GCC countries are migrants, the proportion of spouses is insignificant.

Since the beginning a small segment of migrant women participated in Gulf countries as doctors, nurses and teachers. They are still engaged in such professions. However, due to changes in the demand of labour market, the number of women as principal migrant has increased dramatically. They got employed in newly emerging manufacturing sectors and as domestic workers. Indigenization of certain sectors of job market, local women's increased participation in formal employment, the growth of manufacturing sector are some of the reasons that led to creation of demands for women specific jobs.

The number of such workers increased in such a manner that resulted in feminization of international labour force of some of the labour sending countries. A distinct feature of international migration of Asian women is marriage migration. In the 1970s international marriages mainly took place between western men and Asian women. Since the rise of inter- regional migration, international marriages are increasingly taking place between persons of various Asian countries. Japan, Taiwan, South Korea and Singapore have witnessed record number of international marriages over the last decade. 9.9 percent of the total marriages of South Korea involve a foreign wife. There is a major demand for health professionals in both western and Asian countries. The U.S. alone requires 1.2 million new and replacement nurses by 2014.

In the developed west one in every 11 person will be over 80 years of age soon. Those countries will require employing a huge number of care givers for the elderly persons. However in some of the developed countries enrolment in nursing education has reduced drastically.

Demand for health professionals is not restricted only to the west. Some of the South East Asian countries like Singapore, Bangkok and Malaysia have developed high quality health services, with the aim of selling health tourism. They also required a large number of nurses every year. Understanding the importance and scope of migration of health workers, some of the Asian countries have liberalized the education system and supported growth of public and private sector training institutions to produce huge number of nurses.

The number of nurses training institutions in the Philippines has grown from 30 to 400. The Philippines, Sri Lanka and India have become major sending countries of nurses. They are sending nurses to the west as well as to other Asian countries. In the following section nature and extent of womens' participation in the short term labour market in Asia has been discussed.

Number

Asia includes some of the major labour sending countries of the world. These are the Philippines, Indonesia, Cambodia, Laos, Myanmar, India, Pakistan, Bangladesh, Nepal and Sri Lanka. Afghanistan has gradually joined in the market. Some of these countries proactively pursue female migration while some others restrict them. In 2006 Nepal sent 178,072 workers overseas. Less then 1 percent of them were women. In 2007 Bangladesh sent 832,609 workers, only 5 percent of them were women. India only recorded migration information of low skilled workers, going to 17 countries.

Again workers, who studied more than Grade 10, also do not need to take clearance from the government agencies. So information on a large number of migrants is missing. Nonetheless available data shows that out of 454,628 Indian workers only 0.05 percent were women. Pakistan sent 183,891 workers of which 0.04 percent was women. In sharp contrast to its other South Asian counterparts 52% of Sri Lankan migrants of 2006 were women. This is a decrease in number of female domestic workers in Sri Lanka. At one point of time 90% of its migrant workers used to be women. Philippines sent 1 million workers in 2006. 60% of them were women. It is estimated with regular and irregular combined 80% of Indonesian workers are women (Asis 2006).

COUNTRIES OF DESTINATION

Asia contains both destination and source countries of migrants. Saudi Arabia, Kuwait, UAE, Qatar, Bahrain, Oman are some of the current major labour receiving countries of the Gulf. South Korea, Hong Kong, Taiwan, Singapore, Malaysia and Thailand are some of the major destination countries of South East and East Asia. Japan is not a typical contract labour receiving country yet it takes women workers under entertainment professions. Some twenty years ago countries like Malaysia and Thailand used to be migrant sending countries. Currently they are both sending and receiving countries.

Therefore it is difficult to compartmentalize countries as sending and receiving. Within South Asia, the Maldives is the only country which formally receives workers. Mauritius on the border of Africa and is another country which receives labour from Asia. It is interesting to observe that labour markets of these Asian countries do not remain static. Moreover, the sending countries compete with each other.

For example India and Pakistan used to be the forerunners as male labour senders to the Gulf. Later Bangladesh entered the market by offering lower wages. In the early 1980s, when Sri Lanka and Indonesia wanted to enter the market, it was difficult for them to capture the male migrant markets. Therefore, strategically they chose the female labour market. Népal only entered the market only in the late 1990s. It drastically undercut the Bangladeshi male workers market by offering even lower wage.

The receiving countries also like to rotate its labour intake among the source countries for their own benefit. Malaysia is a classic example. It used to take a large number of workers both men and women from Indonesia. To reduce Indonesian migration, during the early 1990s it took large number of workers from Bangladesh. Within a short span of time it became the second largest labour receiving country for Bangladesh.

During the 1996-1997 financial crisis, it stopped taking labour from all the sending countries. After the financial crisis was over, it did not renew its agreement with Bangladesh; rather it took workers from Nepal. Again in 2006 and 2007, it more or less stopped taking workers from Nepal but reopened its market to Bangladesh. In 2007, 200,000 Bangladeshi workers went to Malaysia alone. Thus, it can be argued that women migration is more common in the case of South East Asian countries in comparison with South Asian sending countries. It also shows that destination countries are not static.

Sectors of Employment

At the beginning of contract migration to the Gulf, with the exception of the few in the professional category, all of them were men. A few women participated as doctors, teachers and nurses. Demand for women specific jobs surfaced in the 1980s. Domestic work became the major employment generating sector. Gradually the South East and East Asian countries also started employing women workers in similar professions.

As seen earlier Philippines, Indonesia, Sri Lanka, Cambodia, and Laos are major players in this respect. Indians also work as domestic workers. For example, among the 300,000 domestic workers in Kuwait, the Indians are second highest in number. Officially Nepali women are only allowed to work in formal sectors. However, there are large differences between official and unofficial figures. According to UNIFEM estimate, there are around 70,000 Nepali domestic workers who work abroad.

The Department of Labour and Statistics however recorded that only 161 women migrated abroad from 1985 to 2001 as domestic workers. Gulf countries as well as South East Asian countries have established different manufacturing industries. Garments, electronic assembling are some of the example of such factories.

Women from above sending countries participate in this sector. Entertainment is also an important sector of women's employment. However, the Philippines is the major country which participates in this sector. Japan and South Korea are two major destinations.

Recently restrictions have been imposed by the South Korean Government on migration of entertainers to that country. Participation in this sector from South Asia is nominal. This is not to say that women do not migrate from South Asia as entertainers, however, if they do, they do so through informal channels and are thus not reflected in the official figures. Nursing and care giving to the elderly are other important professions where women participate. Philippines, India, Sri Lanka are the major sending countries. Nursing is considered to be one of the safest jobs for women migrants. Pakistan and Bangladesh also sent nurses but in low numbers.

Level of Education

A major difference is observed among the domestic workers of the Philippines and Sri Lanka with other South Asian countries. Educational level of Sri Lankan domestic worker is much higher in comparison with others. All of them are literate, significant portion of them passed school finals. According to Perera 2001, 20% of the Sri Lankan migrants had received primary, 45% secondary and 25% of them had tertiary education.

In case of Nepal and Bangladesh more than 80% of them are either not literate or received some elementary schooling. One can say, demand of workers in certain sector is the single most important factor in bringing the Asian women in the international labour market. Along with the Gulf, South East and East Asia are major destination countries. Women are also working in North America and Western European countries. Women from Asia migrate at a very early age.

Marital Status

Differences are observed in case of marital status among South and South East Asian women migrants. Half of the South Asian women migrants are married. In case of Bangladesh, this is very much shaped by the Bangladesh government policy. As for quite a while only married women were allowed to migrate. In case of Nepal as well majority women who opted for foreign employment were married and some with children. A significant portion of Sri Lankan women workers are unmarried. Proportion of unmarried women during first migration is higher in case of the Philippines and Indonesia.

Remittances of Women Migrants

Over the last decade, remittances have become increasingly prominent, remittance flow to developing countries are estimated to have reached US 240 billion in 2007. This amount; however reflect only transfer through official channels. The true size of remittances received should be much higher. Studies in Bangladesh, Sri Lanka, Philippines, Indonesia show that compared to men women migrant sent larger portion of their remittances.

As seen earlier majority of the female workers are domestic workers. Their food and lodging are mostly taken care of by their employers. They also do not feel secure to keep their earning in the destination country. Therefore they sent almost all of their earning to their home countries. Remittances of female migrants helped many of their families to come out of poverty. Studies found that more than half of female remittances were used for daily consumption, health care and children educations.

Household surveys in El Salvador and Sri Lanka find that children of remittance recipient households have a lower school drop out ratio. In Bangladesh and Sri Lanka these household spent more on private tuition of their children. In Sri Lanka the children in remittance receiving households have higher birth weight, reflecting that remittance enabled households to effort better healthcare. Remittance also provided decent livelihood to other members of their families. Along with strong obligation towards own and extended family some of them are conscious about their future and save a portion of the remittance by keeping them in bank or purchasing insurance and investment bonds. All of these have a high social and economic return.

A striking example of effects of remittance on poverty reduction comes from Nepal where the poverty had ratio has declined by 11 percentage points from 1995 to 2004. Since women migrants are absent, remittance are usually utilized by the family. If migrants are married their remittances are used by their husbands and if they are unmarried, these are used by the parents or elder siblings. Due to lack of opportunists as well as lack information on available avenues for investment women migrants can hardly keep control over their remittances.

However women developed their own mechanisms of saving for future during subsequent migration. Bank and Non bank financial institutions of Asian sending countries are yet to come up with gender sensitive investment opportunists. Along with remittances, skills, ideas, attitudes, knowledge and independent decision making capacity are other positive aspects of female migration.

These are termed as social remittances. Migrant's women knowledge brings positive result in her household and community in many ways. According to UNFPA (2006) such knowledge leads to improved state of family health. The nature of female migration from Asia is to some extent determined by their government policies. In the following section female migration policies of some selected countries are discussed.

SRI LANKA

Sri Lanka can be termed as pioneer in labour migration of women in South Asia. As early as late 1970s its government developed policies to encourage migration of women to Middle East for taking up employment. During the same time large scale internal migration of women was also encouraged through establishment of Export Processing Zones in different urban outskirts of the country. Within a short span of time Sri Lanka became a major player in the Gulf labour market of women workers. By the mid 1980s, 90% of its international labour force became women. It is interesting to note that when Sri Lanka entered into the international labour market the market for male workers was already saturated.

India, Pakistan and Bangladesh were strongly present there. Besides, the construction boom for the time being was over. So, demand for male workers was shrinking. But there existed a major demand for women in domestic and manufacturing sectors. Sri Lanka concentrated on the female labour market. Over a period of 15 years it consolidated its presence in Gulf, expanded to South East Asia as well as to Europe and North America. Since 2000 Sri Lanka has changed its policy and along with female market it planed to enter the male market as well. The second construction boom is witnessed in some countries of Gulf and South East Asia. Now Sri Lanka is also sending a large number of male workers as well.

The number of female workers in comparison to males is reducing since then. Last year 52% of the total migrant force was women in comparison to early 1980s when 90 % of the workers were women. Realising the demand for female labour migrant the Sri Lankan government actively pursued a policy of promoting female labour migration. This was pursued despite opposition of a section of the civil society of Sri Lanka. Now that Sri Lanka has consolidated its presence, the state has become more interested in pursuing male labour migration. This highlights the patriarchal ideology of Sri Lankan State.

BANGLADESH

In early 1981, a Presidential Order barred women workers of semi-skilled and unskilled categories from overseas employment on the ground to protect their dignity abroad. The order was in response to strong demand of the then association of Bangladeshi migrant workers in Kuwait for banning women from migrating. In 1988, government revised its position by replacing the ban with restriction on migration of unskilled and semi-skilled women.

But then in late 1997, an almost complete ban was again imposed on migration of all categories of women except those who were highly qualified professionals such as doctors, engineers and teachers. This was greeted with massive opposition by various sections of civil society: women's organizations, labour organizations, professional groups, chambers of commerce, think-tanks etc. They argued that it is unconstitutional and discriminatory against women, and claimed that it would contribute to trafficking of women.

As a result, government lifted the ban on migration of all other categories of women workers, except domestic workers. In the year 2003 the ministry further eased the restriction by putting an age bar. Unskilled or semi skilled women are allowed to migrate under special permission once they become 25. The impact of above policy change was experienced straight away. Women constituted less than 1% of the annual labour flow since 1991 to 2003.

In 2006, 5% of the total migrant labour force of Bangladesh was women. In 2007 a new government came into power. It took a major stand against malpractices in the recruitment sector of Bangladesh. It dissolved the then Executive Committee of Bangladesh Association of International Recruiting Agencies (BAIRA). Strong monitoring at the airport was established, fresh negotiations were held with the governments of the receiving countries.

As a result compared to 2005, the number of migrants going overseas more than doubled.

NEPAL

When labour migration from Nepal to the Gulf and then to South East Asia and East Asia began in the mid-1990s, women also started participating in the flow. Nepali law allowed labour migration of women subject to permission of guardian. But in March 1998, government imposed a ban on labour migration of women to the Gulf. This happened after the death of Kani Sherpa, a Nepali migrant domestic worker in Kuwait. Sexual violence against Kani Sherpa by her employer and his friends, and ultimately her alleged murder by the employer created a major social outcry. This ultimately led to the government ban.

After continuous campaign by different sections of civil society like women's groups, labour organizations, NGOs, international agencies, media and academia, the ban was finally lifted in January 2003. However, lifting ban only applies to the organized sectors (manufacturing), although it is in the informal sector and particularly in domestic work that the majority of Nepali women have scope of employment. This obstructive policy environment is endangering women migrants of Nepal. The approach of securing women abroad through restricted emigration has proved useless.

It has neither been able to curb migration nor secure women. Because, on one hand, there is large demand for cheap Nepali domestic workers in the receiving countries, particularly in the Gulf; on the other hand, lack of economic opportunities and rising insecurity in Nepal is forcing women to earn a livelihood abroad. But since the policy environment is not in favour of their migration, women are forced to migrate in irregular means. Thus they become more vulnerable during and after migration. Sometimes, recruiters take advantage of the women's vulnerability to fulfill their evil desires. The women sometimes fall pray to traffickers disguised as recruiters and end up in involuntary sex work in destination.

Wage

Problems regarding payment of wage are among the most pervasive ones for women migrants of most of the countries. Paying wages lower than promised is one of the most frequent breaches of contract for them. In Sri Lanka, bulk of whose labour migrants are women domestic workers, non-payment of agreed wages is one of the major complaints of women migrant workers. In 2003, about 20% women workers raised this allegation with the conciliation division of SLBFE. However, the trend seems to be declining as the number of cases reduced from 2,089 in 2002 to 1,437 in 2003. An important study of women migrant workers from Bangladesh has also revealed similar instances. On an average, the wage that women migrants received was 20% lower than the contract wage.

Even signing of contract do not guarantee protection. But the picture is also not very different for the employees of formal sectors like manufacturing and service industries. Wage payment situation is equally depressing for Nepali women migrant workers. For example, the Nepali domestic workers in Hong Kong receive only 60% of their salary stipulated by the law. This is the state of affairs in Hong Kong that is increasingly becoming popular destination with Nepali domestic workers for better work condition. Situation in the Middle Eastern countries is reported to be much worse.

Benefits

Payment of other monetary benefits like overtime and bonus are not much relevant for women workers who work outside industrial sectors. A recent study show that Sri Lankan women garment workers employed in some of the garments hub of the Middle East like Dubai (UAE) and Amman (Jordan) earn more in terms of overtime than basic wage. Overtime payments can go upto nearly 50% of total monthly earning. But not all are so fortunate. Some of the Bangladeshi garment workers who worked in UAE reported irregular overtime payments. Domestic workers of Bahrain, Kuwait, Lebanon and UAE do not receive any overtime payment (ILO 2004).

Working Hours

Working hours is another major aspect of work condition. Long or overstretched working hours is an experience commonly shared by Asian migrant women by and large. Although it is a problem in case of both domestic work and factory work, the degree is much sharper in the former than the later. Heavy workload ranging from 15 to 20 hours a day is frequent among women domestic workers.

Studies on Bahrain, Kuwait, Lebanon and UAE show that average working hours of domestic workers per week is over 100 hours which is more than double of standard 40/48 hours per week. One micro study has 54% Sri Lankan domestic workers employed in the Gulf reporting 18 to 20 hours work day. Even among women migrant workers from Bangladesh, domestic workers are the most vulnerable group with regard to working hours. Three-fourths of them, all employed in the Gulf worked 15 to 18 hours a day.

This again would increase further during the Islamic holy month of Ramadan as the adults of the household did not go to bed before taking their *Sehris* (early morning meals). After going to bed at the last leg of night, the domestic workers had to wake up at early next morning to attend the minors and the elders.

Holidays

Weekly holidays and leave are necessary for refreshing one's work performance. But women workers do not get them on a regular basis, even though they are entitled to. Women are no exception. However, this does not seem to be a common trend. Studies covering Sri Lankan migrant women haven't given much attention to this aspect. Nearly 88% domestic workers could not have regular weekly holidays. They were not aware of this entitlement. Another 8% were not allowed to enjoy weekly holidays although they were aware of it.

Situation of industrial workers are however much better. More than 57% Bangladeshi women factory workers in the

Middle East had at least one weekly holiday. Filipino workers who have taken up work outside the Gulf like in Hong Kong, Korea and the European countries are relatively better off in this regard. Because labour laws are more articulated in those countries and their implementation is closely monitored. Singapore also strictly followed regarding weekly holidays. Those working in Lebanon, Kuwait and Bahrain got just one or two days off a month (ILO 2004).

Food and Accommodation

Domestic workers have to eat and live with the employers in general. Employers usually organized accommodation for the factory workers. Small proportion of Sri Lankan domestic workers reported that they had problems with poor quality of food or were denied food as a form of punishment. Likewise, 5% of them had poor accommodation. The factory workers on the other hand, mostly in garments, were in general satisfied with their food and accommodation. Most Bangladeshi workers, whether employed in factory or home, initially had problems to adjust with Middle Eastern food. Some domestic workers had other problems as well like given insufficient food and served with stale food. On the contrary, some had abundant food to their disposal and there were employers who bought items that allowed the migrant workers to cook their own food.

Workplace Conditions

In the Gulf women factory workers found factory temperature intolerably hot. Therefore, it is very hard for someone unused to such condition to work there. Workplace temperature is particularly crucial for Bangladeshi workers as they are from moderate climate region (neither too hot nor too cold). One research on factory worker in Middle Eastern countries shows that factories had sufficient sanitation facilities. Access to clean drinking water also did seem to be of little problem with most women workers. Little less than half of them could drink filtered water and about half of them had to drink supply water. With regard to safety arrangements, factories mostly had emergency fire exits. But more than 88% women workers reported that access to those exits were so inconvenient that they would not be of much help during fire.

Freedom of Movements

Domestic workers working in Bahrain, Kuwait, Lebanon and UAE reported that their freedom of movement was controlled. These included lack of access to telephone, control over receiving and/or sending correspondence, and social isolation from other domestic workers or friends. According to ILO (2004) around 50% domestic workers in Kuwait, Bahrain and UAE alleged physical, verbal or sexual abuse. Such instances were much lower (37%) in Lebanon.

Sexual abuse was mostly perpetrated by employers (sponsors) as well as their sons or other men visiting (ILO 2004). Because domestic work involves individualized work condition, isolation from other workers, least likelihood of establishing networks, absence of social protection, lack of legal recognition as work leading to lack of legal protection as a worker etc. A section of domestic workers are irregular in status. They work in a private sphere without contract. Without legal protections do not report abuses they are subjected to fearing loss of job.

Abuses

Approximately 10% of the women migrant workers from Sri Lanka have harassment and abuse as serious problem. However, it is difficult to measure the extent of 'harassment' since it is not defined. But it continues to form a considerable proportion of the complaints lodged by women migrants, domestic workers in particular. While in 2002, approximately 17% complaints of domestic workers were of harassment, it was nearly 20% in 1996. Another estimate found rate of verbal abuse, physical abuse and sexual harassment respectively as 6%, 9% and 20% among domestic workers.

On an average 24.5% of Bangladeshi women factory workers in the Middle East, mostly garment employees have reported verbal abuse by supervisors and fellow workers. Nepali women migrants have also experienced verbal, physical and sexual abuse. Any statistics on their extent is hardly available. However, cases of such sufferings, particularly from the Middle East are frequently reported in Nepalese media.

Healthcare

Labour laws of the Middle Eastern countries in general require employers to provide health and safety insurance for migrant workers. However, this excludes several categories of workers including domestic workers. Therefore, in many cases domestic workers have to pay for their own healthcare that is often quite expensive from their limited earning. Despite that their access to healthcare is not ensured, as some employers might not allow them to seek such facility when it is required.

Social Protection

Most of the receiving countries of women migrant workers offer limited protection to them. The reality of these countries involve existence of laws discriminatory in terms of gender, race and citizenship; insufficient legal recognition, lack of legal protection, inadequate access to legal support, ineffective enforcement of law etc. Only 57% domestic workers in Kuwait have health and social security coverage. Those from Bahrain, Lebanon and UAE were not privilege of any such provision. Studies also reveal that system for addressing foreign workers' complaints is inadequate or non-existent in Bahrain, Kuwait, Lebanon and UAE. Running away from the employer's household is illegal and punishable. That will result in police search with the runaway worker's photograph published in local newspapers.

Any person who hides or protects her is also considered to be an offender. When found, she is imprisoned and then deported. If the worker decides to go back home or is going to be deported, she still needs to retrieve her passport from her employer. In some cases, the employer return the passport in exchange of non- payment of due wages. In addition, domestic workers fleeing or running away from exploitative working conditions are subjected to inhuman treatment in the hands of the authorities who treat them as criminals. Although these problems are high in the Middle Eastern countries, they are also evident in South East and East Asian countries to considerable degree. Improvements have been noted in some cases. For example, UAE has issued a new law in May 2001 requiring agents to put cash funds in some banks to insure the increasing cases of wage decrease.

Bahrain is reviewing its labour laws and making its sponsorship laws more flexible wherein change of employers is permitted. On 26 March 2003, the government announced a national plan to assist abused workers in emergency cases. The plan includes temporary shelters or "safe houses", a help hotline and a variety of other measures to which expatriate workers, especially domestic workers, can resort to in case of harassment by their employers. The plan also includes the issuing of a rights and duties manual for those intending to work in Bahrain and a simplified guide to be distributed in embassies, recruitment officers and points of entry to Bahrain. Jordan has recently introduced an amendment concerning registration of recruiting agencies. It allows the ministry of labour to monitor the work of these agencies and take actions against them if they violate the regulations aiming at protecting migrant workers.

The country has also introduced the system of "Special Working Contract for Non-Jordanian Domestic Workers" with support of UNIFEM and ILO. While Jordan's labour law does not include any protection of domestic workers, under this arrangement, migrant domestic workers will be treated in compliance with international human rights standards. It provides with limiting fraud of illegitimate contracts, life insurance, medical care, a designated day off a week, rest days, repatriation upon expiration of the contract, legal minimum wage and equal salaries to Jordanians performing the same work.

Lebanon has created a computerized databank that records the entries of all migrant workers with the names and addresses of their employers/sponsors. It will enable to trace the employers in case of misdeeds. The Lebanese government has also established a complaint procedure. However, this system is not giving satisfactory results due to following reasons: lack of trust in the system, lack of information about complaint procedures and serving the interests of employer. Most recently, the government has instituted a US$1,000 bond on registration of sponsorship to be lodged by the individual employer with the Central Housing Bank.

The bond is intended to cover the air ticket of runaway domestic workers and other contingencies in case of grievances presented by the worker. But this system is criticized as some employers/sponsors who want to avoid its payment resort more often now than before to undocumented workers who even suffer from a larger number of abuses than documented workers (ILO 2004).

Proactive Protection Measures in Sending Countries

Sri Lanka took several institutional measures to protect its women worker. Pre-departure skill and awareness trainings, compulsory registration in SLBFE, free insurance coverage, provision for pension scheme, low interest pre departure loans, low interest housing loans, scholarship for women migrant children, distribution of school books and equipments, organizing health camps for left behind family members are some of the incentives used by the government. Sri Lanka is also largely successful in ensuring protection at destination countries by signing MOUs and ratifying relevant international conventions on migration including the 1990 UN Convention on protection of all migrant workers and their families.

In order to ensure that women's migration endeavour was a safe one, the government of Bangladesh has put certain conditions of protection. The security deposit of the recruiting agents who wish to send women was increased to Bangladeshi

Tk. 5 million. In addition, the government also encouraged the private sector to develop training centres for providing specialized professional skill, communication skill and awareness training to the female migrants. Three such centres were been set up under private initiative. Aspirant women were trained on the use of domestic appliances, taught basic.

These sending countries constitutionally guarantee equality of opportunity for work and freedom of movement to their citizens of both sexes, yet many of them, through promulgation of laws and circulars, from time to time, they have imposed restrictions on such movements of women for international migration. This mindset of state of putting restrictions on women's migration is derived from traditional patriarchal notion of honour and dishonor of family and state associated with control over women's mobility. Sri Lanka is a classic example. Due to economic necessity it developed proactive policy to encourage its women to migrate. Now that it has strongly established itself in the global labour market it has changed its tone and does not proactively look for job markets for their women. Rather, it is now exploring new markets for men.

This highlights the double standard of state. When necessary, it pursued migration of its women. Now that women migration is no longer crucial to its immediate economic well being, it is reverting to traditional ideology men as principal bread earners. Sending country governments should acknowledge the reality of feminization of international migration. Instead of enacting laws that restrict movement of women for work, adequate information should be made available so that aspirant women migrants can make an informed choice.

Women's Participation and Gender Equity

Traditionally men were perceived as bread earners and women were seen in their reproductive roles. Globalization has created opportunities for women's participation in certain types of factory work both inside and outside the country which require women to move. This has definitely complicated traditional patriarchal division of work and space as public and private. In Asia everywhere women move internally and internationally to take up employment. This does challenge the traditional notion of men being the bread winner. International migration, no matter how exploitative it may be has successfully established women's role as principal earners. Again, in many cases male counterpart of women migrants agree to women's migration, jointly accumulate resources as they see cost of women's migration is lower and job opportunities for women are higher. This has ensured the participation of men in power sharing dialogues with their female counterparts.

Gendered Division of Labour within Households

Studies on left behind families indicate that when men migrate women take over double responsibility and successfully perform the house hold functions. However, when a woman migrates a section of the husbands do become more careful children's upbringing and education. They never take up gender specific roles in household maintenance. In the Asian context, the extended family takes over some of the tasks which used to be performed by the woman migrant.

Role of Women in Family Decision- making

Some of the studies on the consequences of migration highlighted that particularly upon return; some women had difficulties in maintaining their newly acquired power in family decision making. This has lead to conflict between husband and wife, father and daughter or sister and brother when women asserted their position in family decision making. The same studies show that a large number of women could retain their share of authority over family decision making through using their negotiating skills which they developed during staying outside the hierarchical family structure. Researchers appreciate that there are marked differences between the woman who departs for migration and the one who returns from it. Therefore, the outcome of migration on gender relationships is not homogenous. Though Asia is the second largest migrant producing region of the world, it produces the least number of female migrants. The female migrant labour force does not constitute more than 5 percent in any of the South Asian states other than Sri Lanka. Domestic work constitutes the most important occupation of the migrant work force, followed by employment in manufacturing sector. Feminization of international labour force has taken place in some of the South East Asian labour sending countries that include Indonesia and the Philippines. Almost one half of Cambodian migrants are also women. Four distinct forms of female migration is visible in Asia.

These are migration of women as dependent spouses, migration of professional workers, temporary contract migration of skilled and low skilled workers and migration through international marriage. This chapter mostly highlighted the trends of skilled and low skilled women workers who are temporarily working mostly within Asia as contract workers. The chapter highlights primacy of temporary labour migration over permanent migration since the early 1970s. It underscored the increasing prominence of Asia as work destination. It demonstrated that Middle Eastern countries created job opportunists for both men and women of different Asian countries. Since 1990s the singular importance of the Gulf region as receiving country in Asia has declined. Some of the South East Asian and East Asian growth economies have also emerged as labour receiving countries. During the initial phase work opportunities were mostly created for men.

Since the 1980s some jobs emerged in the market which created scope for female migration. The demands for female specific job have resulted in feminization of international workforce of some of the labour sending countries. Both Middle East and South East Asian countries required women's labour as service worker, particularly domestic workers as well as in manufacturing sectors. International labour migrants have been identified by ILO as the most vulnerable section of international work force. Compared to men women migrants are more vulnerable. Like their male counterparts the women migrants experience confiscation of travel documents, withholding and non- payment of salary or salary reduction, harsh working conditions, lack of freedom of movements and communication etc. In addition, verbal, physical and sexual abuse is an issue that a section of women migrants have to face. Individual countries through bilateral negotiation attempt to resolve these problems.

A common stand of sending countries regarding the rights of migrant workers in general and female migrants in particular is yet to emerge. The only example of agreement between two sending countries has been between Philippines and Indonesia. Over the last 30 years labour sending countries of Asia has developed their own policies, programmes and institutional structure to govern labour migration. Philippines have become a model for other countries in these respects. In case of governing female migration both Philippines and Sri Lanka have come up with innovative programmes that of mandatory 15 days to 1 month pre-departure training. India and Philippines have achieved major successes in the area of quality training of nurses.

This has resulted in increasing the number of skilled migrants and therefore reducing labour exploitation and increasing remittance. However there is very little inter-governmental initiative to systemically learn from each other. Sending countries can gain immensely from the experience of these countries Female labour migration is a complex process and it involves a number of parties: governments, recruiting agencies, employers and money transfer institutions. A migrant woman also need to know the socio-cultural environment of the destination countries, work conditions, procedures of sending remittance and opportunities available for investment of migrant remittance. She also requires information on all the above issues. Recently, in Bangladesh a media campaign has been launched under which television plays and talk shows, display of messages through bill boards, mega signs, public service announcements through television and radio have been organized.

At the same time for grass roots activation Migrants Rights Protection Committees have been established in some migration intensity districts of the country. This model may be taken up by other South Asian countries for raising awareness about various aspects of migration, including those of female migrants. The Philippines and Sri Lanka have developed some institutional capacities to provide protection to female workers in the destination countries. The other South Asian countries may follow the two examples and establish easy access hotlines and shelter homes for female workers who have difficulties with employers. They may also consider providing legal assistance to female migrants who have work and legal status problems. In some destination countries women workers go through periodic mandatory pregnancy tests.

If they are found to be positive they are sent back home or have to abort. Provision for reproductive and mental health care services to the migrant women in the countries of destination needs to be facilitated. In Asian countries policy played a major role in determining the nature of migration. Being a late entrant in international labour market Sri Lanka accessed it through sending female migrants. The Philippines has also played a proactive policy in ensuring market of female workers. As India, Bangladesh and Nepal imposed bans and restrictions on female labour migration from time to time the number of females in the stock of international migrants is relatively low.

It is perhaps due to this factor that these countries have experienced flow of women through irregular channels. Most Asian states send female migrants to provide services at the low end of care giving sector, India being the exception that sends highly skilled nurses. There is a burgeoning demand for nurses in global market. Demand will rise in the Gulf states as well as developed countries of the world including North

America and Europe. A major problem in accessing the market is the quality of nursing training that exists. The other South Asian countries may consider uplifting their training standard by establishing links with the Indian training institutions. National data on migration is collated differently by state agencies of various SAARC countries.

The absence of standard data hinders quality comparative research. The Task Force will encourage states to agree to a set of common indicators that may be developed by concerned experts and demographers so that there is consistency and standardization in migration data. The paper found that there is a similarity of problems that the Asian countries face in migration governance. Each of the countries has attempted to address the problems in their own ways. This chapter strongly argues periodic sharing of experiences among the sending countries of Asia to learn from each others experience. This will also help reducing unhealthy competition among these countries.

3

Urbanisation and Gender Struggle

Urbanisation has been one of the salient features of social change across the world in modern times. Cities and conurbations are where different cultures and social developments such as globalization and exploitation of human and natural resources converge. At the same time, cities provide the space where historically and culturally varied constellations of gender relations have been recorded. New cultures also rapidly emerge across various urban subgroups. In most of the developing world, institutions are implicitly shaped by a patriarchal ideology. Accordingly, gender construction is tied to value and belief systems that undermine women, exposing the more deprived to poverty, sexual discrimination, abuse and their consequences.

Women and girls are doubly marginalized, because of gender and the physical and social conditions of the poor. But on top of this, with its focus on the physical and spatial aspects of development, urban planning disregards the unique, gender-differentiated situation of women. The major challenge is to determine the extent to which evolving cultural trends advance women's role in the development of human settlements.

Women make up nearly half of the international migrant population (UNFPA 2003). Gender differences in the proportions of male/female migrants to urban areas are obviously determined by certain cultural factors in the place of origin.

These include lack of equal access to, rights in, and control over, economic resources, such as land. Benschop (2002) notes that "as compared to rural areas, women in cities and towns tend to have more access to land and housing; women, more often than not, 'own' shacks or structures in informal settlements or rent a house or room."

These factors give women some of the autonomy which cultural factors deny them in rural areas. Examples from Latin America suggest that the scale and nature of migration into urban areas is largely influenced by three types of factors: first, decisions in rural households about who should migrate and why; second, constraints placed by households on women's work outside the home; and, third, demand for female labour in urban areas.

Evidence shows that in some regions, their traditional reproductive and productive roles in rural areas do not prevent women from moving to urban settlements. For example, in Eastern Europe, Latin America and the Caribbean, the overall ratio of women to men is higher in urban than in rural areas, and the reverse is true for Africa and Asia.

HOUSEHOLD RELATIONS AND GENDER ROLE TRANSFORMATION

FAMILY INSTITUTION IN TRANSITION

Across cultures, the family is the basic social structure most likely to meet individual needs and expectations. Women typically spend much more time in the house than men as they perform their reproductive and household roles. This imbalance has implications on poor urban women, especially as the structure of the family unit is changing and female-headed households are on the increase. Traditional sociology links the family institution to blood and marriage ties but modernization and Urbanisation are changing all this.

The initial dramatic shift from extended to nuclear family only paved the way for alternative forms: single-parent, step-parent and blended households, remarriages and cohabitation with children. Children's homes, foster homes and shelters for the homeless are other emerging forms of families. Institutional families act as safe landing pads for orphaned, abused and neglected children. In addition, more and more gay couples are raising children under emerging legislation.

These cultural transformations affect mostly poor urban women. There are more households headed by a female than a male single parent (UNDP, Human Development Reports 1995, 2002, 2003). Divorce, separation, cohabitation and re-marriage place peculiar strains on women's social and economic lives. Such changes and the attendant social problems trigger different policy responses across regions, depending on context.

More specifically, responses are a function of how citizens and politicians experience and perceive change, define new social issues associated with it, understand the range of choices open to them and interpret their interests within that range.

GENDER RELATIONS, ROLES AND RESPONSIBILITIES IN THE CONTEXT OF URBANISATION

In the developing world, women migrate from the countryside to urban areas for many reasons, but they always expect a better life. What they often find instead is drudgery and dire poverty, without hope for improvement. In urban slums and shanty settlements, women bear the burden of raising children in the most difficult circumstances. They are under constant threat of eviction, without a secure home for themselves and their families. They endure the indignities and dangers of unhygienic toilets, shared by hundreds; they are the most vulnerable to crime and violence, and are inordinately affected by the HIV/AIDS pandemic, as both victims and caregivers.

Some 25 per cent of the world's households have women as their heads, and in urban areas (especially in Latin America and Africa) that proportion can exceed 50 per cent. Women typically represent a high proportion of those in informal settlements worldwide, and they are among the poorest. The growth in female-headed households is often equated with the growth in poor or disadvantaged households, but female headship can have positive aspects.

Female-headed households are likely to be less constrained by patriarchal authority and female heads may experience greater self- esteem, more personal freedom, more flexibility to take on paid work, better control over finances, and little or no physical or emotional abuse. Female heads may be empowered insofar as they are better able to further both their personal interests in education and business and the well-being of their dependants. In Africa, the majority of urban farmers are women, mainly from female-headed households. The case study below illustrates how some women in cities try to survive and feed their families.

CASE STUDY 1- URBAN AGRICULTURE, KENYA

In Kenya, home-grown food is critical to the nutritional status of families: 25 per cent of urban families in the six major cities claim they cannot survive without self-produced food; 56 per cent of urban farmers are female but the ratio rises to 62 per cent in the larger cities, and 64 per cent of women farmers are from female-headed households, showing how critical urban agriculture is to the survival of poor families. Urban farmers are not recent migrants.

Pressure is such that new arrivals have less access to land than longer-term residents. A large proportion of urban farmers are white-collar workers, even mid-level bureaucrats, with larger house plots. A critical issue for urban development is land ownership or user rights, as modern systems of land registration clash with inherited patterns. In Kenya, only 41 per cent of urban farmers own the land they use and 42 per cent (primarily the poorest) grow their crops on government land.

EMPLOYMENT AND LIVELIHOODS IN URBAN INFORMAL SETTLEMENTS

Gender, Poverty and Income-generation in Informal Settlements

If the lives of urban slum dwellers are to be improved, one must consider how best they can increase their incomes. Through their involvement in urban agriculture, women are vital to the urban economy as small entrepreneurs, traders, workers and providers of food security. The following case study illustrates best practices of women's response to unemployment in the urban informal sector.

CASE STUDY 2- STREET VENDORS IN HANOI, VIETNAM

Hanoi's female vendors team up in groups and some rent and share rooms where they cook and eat together. They also make food for sale, a cheap and convenient service for most urban dwellers. Some provide quick, cheap personal-care services, such as hair-cutting. Relieving urban middle-class working women and housewives of domestic chores earns Hanoi's poor women a living. A survey found that 70 per cent walked from door to door, carrying their goods in a pair of baskets with a pole across their shoulders (47 per cent), in hand or head baskets (15 per cent), or in a trolley (7 per cent). Others (30 per cent) used bicycles and only one a motorcycle.

As for men, 56 per cent used bicycles and the others either a trolley or a toolbox (36 per cent), or worked as taxi drivers (8 per cent). Women mostly lacked fixed sales pitches. Other major complaints were: no place to work or sit, official harassment, thin profits, costly transportation, mistreatment, heavy loads, long walks, no care for children, theft, lack of housing, health, and lack of toilets. They felt there was potential for forming a support network. The disparity is glaring between male and female strategies for survival, and women seem more able to organize around small-scale businesses. But why should women face more transportation hardships than men? Are city planners still foot-dragging over certain gender-responsive issues?

Obviously, in Hanoi, gender-responsive transportation, security, childcare services, and access to sanitation would ease female street-vendors' burden in their struggle for survival. Street vending is the most visible aspect of women's informal business. But this activity is often viewed as a nuisance or obstruction to commerce. For lack of legal status and recognition, women face frequent harassment and eviction from their pitches by competing shopkeepers, as well as confiscation and even arrest. Workplaces are often dirty, dangerous and devoid of basic services. For all these risks, street vending is the only option for many poor people, especially women (WIEGO - undated).

SELF-EMPLOYMENT AND MICRO-ENTERPRISES

The need to recognize women's economic capacity and potential has been a concern for local, national, and international bodies and poverty-reduction strategies. Currently a number of donors are providing support to women's self-employment through micro-enterprise.

CASE STUDY 3 - WOMEN SELF-MOBILIZING FOR EMPLOYMENT IN GUJARAT, INDIA

Gujarat's Shri Mahila Sewa Sahakari Bank was set up in 1974 for poor self-employed women at the initiative of 4,000 of them. Running the bank is a board elected by its 51,000 depositors. On top of finance - linked services Sewa has started a work security insurance scheme and a housing programme. It is now expanding into rural areas through savings and credit groups which channel surpluses into Sewa's development activities. Sewa gives poor women control of natural and financial resources, such as helping them build their own water facilities, such as wells, ponds, hand pumps, etc. Loan recovery rates are high thanks to mutual trust and an understanding of borrowers' individual circumstances. Sewa members skip predatory private money-lenders and gain self-confidence as they develop the skills required to deal with formal organizations. Sewa has broken the vicious circle of indebtedness and dependence on middlemen and traders, and has changed women's bargaining powers for the better.

WOMEN IN EXPORT PROCESSING ZONES

Most developing countries attract foreign investment through export processing zones (EPZs), also known as "special economic" or "free trade" zones. One of the incentives offered is the low cost of the workforce, which the 2003 World Development Report estimates is 70–90 per cent female. The following case study from Indonesia clearly outlines the gender and cultural issues and conflicts which women experience in EPZs.

CASE STUDY 4 - EPZS AND FEMALE WORKERS IN INDONESIA

EPZ female workers typically endure intolerable working conditions and long hours. Indonesia's minimum wage, which ranges up to US$1.84 in some areas, meets only 60 to 70 per cent of the minimum physical needs of a single individual against the backdrop of wide fluctuations in fuel and basic goods prices. Employers often call in the army to deal with strikes but workers are becoming more bold and militant. Females provide the bulk (80 to 95 per cent) of those involved in the actions and are a majority in the bodies elected to lead them.

Typical demands are better pay and working conditions, freedom of association, praying time, gender-specific steps to combat sexual harassment and gender discrimination, together with maternity and menstruation leave as required by existing law. EPZ employers rarely provide the statutory three months' fully paid maternity leave and usually dismiss pregnant women; when allowed to return to work, these lose any seniority and start from the bottom again.

Humiliating material evidence is required for two days' monthly menstruation leave, which if granted entails loss of bonus or two days' wages. Since unions are not allowed in EPZs, there is no institutional collective bargaining. A group of workers, usually organized by non-governmental organizations, takes the initiative and negotiates with management. Any better wages or working conditions thus won benefit only the workers in the factory.

The structural disparities of gendered systems shape female labour issues. The gender allocation of social and economic roles restricts women's access to the means of production (from credit to training opportunities) and confines them to a limited number of occupations and markets. Recognition is growing of women's multiple roles and the value of not only their productive, but also their reproductive contributions.

Longstanding work standards are in question, new forms of labour organizations emerge and the relationship between work and leisure is being recast. Stakeholders in human settlements development will recognize that the economic capacity of women in urban areas is linked to basic services and security of tenure, and that as their economic activities concentrate in the informal economy and close to home, they need those resources that are essential to doing business and working in residential areas.

GENDER, LAND, HOUSING AND PROPERTY RIGHTS

Land and Property Rights

There is a general consensus around the fact that although insecurity of tenure affects millions of people across the world, women face additional risks and deprivation related to culture and gender. In South Asia and Africa, many women are still exposed to discrimination in access to land, shelter and property rights despite policy and legal reforms. The vast majority cannot afford to buy land and some countries do not recognize their equal rights to land. In Africa, comparatively few statutory books entrench women's access to land and property: examples may be found in Burkina Faso, Malawi, Mozambique, Niger, Rwanda, South Africa, Uganda, the United Republic of Tanzania and Zimbabwe. There is no legislation, but no impediment either, in Eritrea and Ethiopia. Botswana, Lesotho and Namibia are currently amending the relevant statutes. In other cases formal law, traditional systems and social norms (including customary and religious law), often deny women the right to acquire and inherit property, particularly in countries where shariah law applies.

It must be noted here that customary tenure is often more dynamic and complex than statutory systems; and for all their restricted access to ownership through inheritance or purchase, women as heads of households may have significant indirect access and rights to use land. But then not all women in such cultures get married, or remain married to ensure their secure tenure. Other factors constraining women's access to land and property ownership include poverty, lack of credit facilities and affordable housing finance, together with low awareness of human and legal rights and poor representation of women in decision-making bodies in charge of administration and management of land and property.

Worse still, women face administrative bottlenecks in land offices, tribunals, and court systems. With the growing consensus that the right to acquire and inherit property is a basic human right applicable equally to men and women, some countries tailor formal and informal tenure arrangements to different local social, political and economic circumstances in order to enable women's access to property. In some countries, affirmation of co-ownership of land has led to the acceptance of women's equal rights to property, whereas others endorse joint ownership of property for legally married couples.

Elsewhere, more or less formal types of consensual unions are understood to embody property rights. Therefore, social movement triggers changes, and equality becomes more widely accepted in social relations. Some countries have eased the constraints on women's control over land and property: in Latin America, the law provides for joint ownership; whereas in Uganda, the other spouse's consent is required before any transfer. In general, legal systems that endorse joint ownership gives women better security of tenure.

Housing

Lack of access and control over housing in informal urban areas is a major problem for women. In some cases, women are discriminated against and at times landlords evict them from their rented rooms for non-payment. For many low-income urban dwellers and particularly women, the situation is such that they lack the resources for adequate shelter. What may be termed "gender blindness" in housing and basic service programmes is becoming increasingly apparent. Low-cost housing or site and service programmes rarely consider the needs and priorities of women in terms of design, infrastructure and services. Women are excluded through eligibility criteria, methods of beneficiary recruitment and cost-recovery mechanisms.

Gender dimensions affect renting and owner-occupation. In Latin America and West Africa, female-headed households are more likely to be tenants or sharers than owners, but in Bangladesh female-headed households and supported households are concentrated in the poorest and potentially most vulnerable housing conditions. There are three main reasons for this: first, women are often excluded from official housing programmes offering owner- occupation; second, female-headed households tend to be poorer and, since poorer households frequently rent, women tend to be tenants; and, third, although most female-headed households lack the time and skills required, lack of funds for professional labour often forces them to build their own housing (UN 1995).

GENDER, VIOLENCE AND FORCED EVICTIONS

Urban poor women and children are particularly affected by forced eviction. More often than not, forced eviction by public authorities, city councils, landlords and agents takes place in informal urban settlements. Human Rights Watch (2003) noted that although all women are vulnerable, divorced or separated women and widows - including AIDS widows - suffer some of the most extreme violations. Divorced and separated women are often left with only the clothes on their backs as their husbands keep the home and other property.

Widows are often evicted from their homes as in-laws rob them of their possessions and invade their homes and lands. These unlawful appropriations happen even more readily when the husband died of AIDS. In some places, widows are forced to undergo customary, sexual practices such as "wife inheritance" or ritual "cleansing" in order to keep their property. Beatings and rape by the evictors have been reported in several countries. The following example from Bangladesh summarizes the brutality of evictions and their lack of regard for human rights.

CASE STUDY 5 - URBAN CLEANSING IN DHAKA, BANGLADESH

Dhaka's population is over 11 million, of which 46.7 per cent live in absolute poverty and about half this group in hard-core poverty. Landlessness, natural disasters, river erosion and lack of income-earning opportunities drive the rural poor to urban areas, especially Dhaka's sprawling slums and squatter settlements. But public authorities do not recognize their rights to live there. Some argue that the urban poor should be taken back to their villages and resettled there, and indeed such a programme is currently being implemented.

When, in August 2001, the Government launched large-scale pull-downs (including settlements upgraded by UNICEF) and evictions, the worst affected were female garment workers, who came back to their sleeping shacks after the shift to find that they were no more. According to non-governmental organizations, some 12,000 families were affected. The Coalition for the Urban Poor (CUP) organized a protest rally, prayers and a high-level seminar to stop the evictions. Non-governmental organizations also showed the communities how to resist eviction threats, to which the Government has finally called a halt.

GENDER, CULTURE AND URBAN GOVERNANCE

GENDER AND URBAN GOVERNANCE

For all their obvious presence as citizens, women, especially when poor, remain under- represented in governing structures, especially local decision-making, owing to social and political gender-related factors. Affirmative action is in order, alongside innovations like the Competition and Awards for gender-responsive, women-friendly cities (in the Latin American and Caribbean and Asian-Pacific regions) as well as grassroots awareness-raising to involve more women in city governance.

Basic services, human rights, economic capacity, transportation, violence and security of tenure are major issues for women who must, therefore, be involved in decisions regarding them. Women are major users of water and their inclusion in water management committees has been found to improve both service and payment levels. Likewise, involving women in planning and management of sanitation improves systems, makes them socially and culturally responsive and enhances communities' sense of ownership.

GATHERING STRENGTH FROM INFORMAL RELATIONSHIPS

The variety and density of housing in informal settlements provide many opportunities for interaction. Often, especially in Africa, poor women form groups for economic purposes (so-called "merry-go-rounds", where group members contribute money for lending to an individual) to sort out their needs (purchase of household items, etc.). Group members also assist each other for funerals, weddings and emergency fundraising. These social support networks re-invent ties beyond kinship and have served as vehicles for campaigns against child abuse and wife-beating.

Development projects can use them as entry points into the community, all the more so as these groups have already identified their leader or leaders, who can then be relied upon when planning for development in informal settlements. Informal relationships are not confined to cities; they extend to rural areas and relatives occasionally trade cash or goods from the city against a constant flow of food from the countryside. This maintains links between the rural and urban areas, which to some extent balance the development process and spread new ideas.

GENDER, HUMAN RIGHTS AND THE COMMERCIAL SEXUAL EXPLOITATION OF WOMEN

PROSTITUTION (COMMERCIAL SEX WORK)

Prostitution has a direct link with the break-up of small-scale communities and the advent of large, anonymous urban areas together with commercialized social relations. In 1985, the International Committee for Prostitutes' Rights demanded that sex workers be guaranteed human rights, including freedom of speech, travel, immigration, work, marriage, motherhood, health, and housing. As part of this rights-based agenda, the sex worker rights movement aims to curb unethical and abusive behaviour towards prostitutes. This includes harassment and extortion by police and other authorities; denial of fair treatment during arrest; imprisonment without due process; failure to investigate or prevent crimes committed against prostitutes (rape, physical violence, murder); and threats and reprisals against sex workers' families.

The purpose here is to draw attention to the needs of those poor urban women involved in prostitution. Although it is almost impossible to eradicate it, governments cannot continue to ignore those involved. They require health, sanitation, housing and security services. Whether prostitution contributes to gross domestic product (GDP) remains a moot point. Either way, it must be seen as another strategy of informal economic sustenance some women have adopted in informal settlements.

CASE STUDY 6 - SEX WORKERS ORGANIZING IN BANGLADESH

Sex workers in developing countries see human rights as a crucial tool to address the double discrimination they face as women and as prostitutes. Women who were evicted from the Tan Bazar brothel in Bangladesh recently won the right to return to their place of work, with local non-governmental organizations' support of their rights and international attention to strengthen their cause. In 1999, when 3,500 sex workers were evicted from Tan Bazar, they and their families were forced to move to a vagrants' shelter where they faced sexual harassment, abuse and extortion. When deciding the case brought by 100 sex workers, the High Court concluded that the Government had no legal grounds to evict the brothel occupants because prostitution, when the basis for women's livelihood, is not illegal.

The case is crucial as it shows that if sex workers' human rights must be upheld, one should look beyond civil and political freedoms and also consider economic and social rights, including the right to work. As Carol Jenkins, an advocate for Bangladeshi sex workers put it: "No other approach but that of human rights - such as the rights of a citizen and the right to work - would have worked in Bangladesh. Because a coalition of over 60 human rights organizations put its strength behind the sex workers' cause, the High Court would hear the case." The challenge remains to raise awareness, strengthen organizations, and train effective lobbyists who can win permanent status for sex workers' rights.

SEX TOURISM

Sex tourism has direct harmful effects on the lives of women and girls. A large majority of the women involved may have done so deliberately and outside any sex slavery and trafficking, but their social and political circumstances (school drop-out, higher rates of illiteracy, disease and poverty) are not alien to their decision. Sex tourism may attract some well-off urban women as well, but the effects of sexually transmitted diseases (STDs), in particular, HIV/AIDS, are visible across all categories, with slums the most affected, including by other infectious diseases. And since the majority of women partaking in sexual tourism are young, globalization takes an even heavier toll.

ROLE OF CULTURE IN HUMAN SETTLEMENTS DEVELOPMENT

Popular Culture and Arts

Cities typically preserve a nation's culture in museums, archives, cultural centres, performing arts and media, providing incomes for young and adult people from informal settlements. There are no reliable data but, in Kenya for instance, female groups take to entertainment as a source of income. Popular culture gives the young opportunities both to consume existing forms and re-invent some.

The contributions they make in the fight against HIV/AIDS, crime, immorality and general social deviance through music, drama and poetry are quite significant. Young people from informal urban settlements (slums, ghettos) have often come to epitomize success in these areas of popular culture. They also inspire others to venture into more positive out-of-school activities than gang behaviour (idling, crime and prostitution). Others have used drama and the visual arts to make effective contributions to the development of informal settlements.

Media

Accessible media like radio and television have been instrumental in lobbying and advocating for the social, economic and reproductive rights of poor women and young people. Locally composed drama brings their daily plight to the attention of policy-makers, highlighting lack of access to basic services, domestic violence and HIV/AIDS. In Kenya, artists from informal settlements appear in popular broadcast programmes. The media widely publicize forced evictions, harassment and their consequences, with rights activists often calling for action. Broadcasts also broach development-related issues regarding health, education and safety. But then what proportion of slum-dwelling women has access to radio or TV? Ownership depends on income. Most males are at an advantage as social clubs provide such media, which further widens the gap for women.

Literature

Reading is another good channel of information but its effectiveness depends on whether people have access to books, magazines, etc. In the past, writers have used literature as a way of telling the world about problems affecting their communities. Where the situation of poor urban women is highlighted either directly or indirectly, they are often stereotyped as prostitutes, or preys to males. Their dwellings when depicted are often poor, with the woman having to depend for extra money from a certain man in order to dress appropriately and pay rent.

However, another brand of authors, typically from West Africa, often portray poor urban women as militants ready to fight for their rights with law enforcers. For instance, So Long a Letter, by the Senegalese novelist Mariama Bâ, explores the gains and losses that two female characters experience through Urbanisation and colonial re-acculturation over their lifetimes. But, here again, poverty means that many women will never benefit from such wisdom, all the more so as libraries in most cities are elitist and charge fees.

Role of Religion

Religion is an integral part of any culture but its influence varies from individual to individual. More women than men subscribe to religion, giving them a common ground to discuss their plight and to take appropriate action. The influence of religion on women's groupings in informal settlements is not well documented. The interrelationship between culture, gender and Urbanisation is a complex one. The poorest of the poor in urban areas are women, all the more so as they remain hostages to patriarchal ideologies. Most cities in the developing world are not women-friendly as discomforts - such as poor transportation - and danger lurk everywhere: lack of employment, housing, basic services - notably water and health - and sexual and physical violence. Urban planning tends to overlook gender issues in access to land, property and housing.

Many countries have reformed law and policies accordingly. But a more holistic and inclusive approach is still required; in particular, reforms of inheritance and marital property regimes and those of laws and policies on land, housing, credit and gender must be consistent between them. Urban and peri-urban land issues must come within national land policy and be linked to rural land issues. Gender must be a cross-cutting perspective, including in budget allocation. Implementation of such laws and policies remains a huge challenge, requiring concerted efforts at all levels if women's rights to land and property are to become realities. Popular culture promoting gender equality and the advancement of women has a role to play.

Tensions are obvious between economic growth, social equity and political legitimacy in cities around the world. Urban governance allows them to coalesce and seek resolution. But it must involve women alongside men, since each gender experiences and uses the urban environment in different ways and has different priorities for urban services and infrastructure. The case studies mentioned in this chapter highlight women's success in informal sector trading, self-help employment through micro financing, lobbying and advocacy, as well as turning culture into an effective tool for development and economic empowerment.

KEY ISSUES FOR DISCUSSION

How best can culture be used to create an urban environment where men and women can live in peace and harmony, as equal human beings, and work in partnership for social justice and development? Why have women activists and women's affairs ministries focused so little on music, art, poetry, dance and drama to further women's rights and economic empowerment? What is the missing link and how should this be addressed? How can poor women in informal settlements manage security of tenure for the land they occupy, and how can this help address the adverse impact of poverty in slums?

Can we keep talking about safer cities without adequately addressing the abhorrent crimes committed against women caught up in prostitution and sex tourism, especially the more vulnerable who are driven into the trade by poverty and gender discrimination? Women predominate in the informal sector, and they also feed the city. How long can authorities continue to disregard the informal sector, dismiss the plight of the urban poor, and condemn women to poverty? Can governments and development agencies reconsider their stance, change policies as required and reduce poverty?

The majority of urban migrants come by themselves or with only their immediate family (spouse and children). This has led to the fragmentation of families and a shift in the composition of the traditional family unit. Even people living in remote rural areas now usually have some family or community linkages to the city. Isolated from extended family, new arrivals to urban areas lack an immediate support network, socially or economically. Single parent families are more common. Children are more often left alone because grandparents, aunts and uncles are not around while parents are working.

Socializing with new and unknown local influences can put both children and adults at increased risk of harm. Urban youth in particular can be exposed to social groups that exploit their poverty and frustration. Criminal gangs or militant groups often recruit from this vast pool of disenfranchised urban youth. Conversely though, the city also creates new opportunities for community that may not previously have been necessary or possible. If people with experiences, livelihoods or challenges in common can find each other in a city, they can form powerful communities to call for change and protection.

THE GENDER DIMENSION

Migrant women need particular protection from the alienation that urban living can bring. At first glance, life in the city brings many benefits to women that traditional rural lifestyles have not offered. They can be economically independent of their families, whether married or unmarried. Young women in Asia are often employed in the garment industry, fish processing and other factories. Even though they earn minimum wages and the industries are not well represented by labour laws, it can still be empowering.

But there is another side to the urban coin. Lack of monitoring of female-dominated workforces leaves girls and women vulnerable to sexual abuse, unfair dismissal and even trafficking. Women from slum areas are more likely to marry early and have more children than women in the rest of the city. Without the extended family of rural settings, women are then challenged to capacity on their ability to care for their children and earn money at the same time.

Lack of access to maternal and child health information and care, as well as family planning resources, can intensify the challenges. Women's urban experiences provide both great opportunities and great risks for addressing poverty. Urban women can easily create communities of support in both their work and home environment, but struggle when they do not know how.

ALTERNATIVE COMMUNITIES

Traditional rural communities form geographically, in clusters of extended family that eventually grow to become villages. With land available, proximity to neighbours is a choice rather than a necessity. In urban settings, however, people settle wherever they can find and afford shelter. In slum communities, often the only element they will have in common with their new neighbours is the urgent need for income. Development in urban settings is still based on community support, but to be effective it must reach out to alternative communities, who may have work, beliefs, cultural practices or causes in common rather than geography.

Finding these alternative communities should not exclude children's communities. Outside school, children gather together as child labourers, rubbish scavengers or beggars. All of these groups can benefit from targeted programmes including informal education, mobile health clinics, drop-in centres or vocational training. The needs of alternative urban communities may also be addressed through the power of information, networks and partnerships. This involves equipping common interest or identity groups with knowledge of their rights, what is available to them, and linking them with potential partners who can advocate with or for the urban poor.

We are leaders and campaigners of urban poor movements in the Philippines, India, Indonesia, and China. We gathered together for a three-day meeting on February 16-18, 2009 to put forward our agenda for social protection, citizenship rights and urban change. We examined the situation of poor urban dwellers living in rapidly urbanizing cities in the Philippines, India, Indonesia, and China and came to the conclusion that poor urban dwellers, many of them women and children, live in abject poverty. We concluded further that we must bring into sharp focus the legitimate claim of poor urban dwellers to a dignified and secure existence in cities by pushing for the right of all urban poor dwellers to efficient public services, participation in urban planning and social protection within the framework of citizenship rights and sustainable and just urban development.

We deplore the continued chaos and misery in Asian cities that is the result of unplanned Urbanisation. Asia's growing Urbanisation has come to represent the worst of urban poverty and inequality. Tens of millions are currently living in miserable conditions in cities across Asia without adequate jobs and access to public services like water, healthcare, electricity, transport, and education. Everyday, one million people flock to Asian cities, fueling the growth of these cities but also further swelling the ranks of the poor.

We are these poor people. We are called many names: urban poor, slum dwellers, migrant workers, among others. We come to the city to seek opportunities for employment and fulfillment but we are condemned to live in slums, on sidewalks and in subways, under bridges, or in decrepit tenements, fighting social exclusion and dodging the perils of hunger and urban violence on a daily basis. Now that urban-based industries are feeling the crunch of the global financial crisis, the resulting job cuts are hitting us first and hardest, pushing us farther beyond the margins of desperation and uncertainty. It is time we speak out. We are tired of being ignored for what we really are and regarded only as blight - thorny problems that cities must get rid of to pave the way for more development.

We want to say these:

- We are urban dwellers. We are all inhabitants of the cities we live in. The city belongs to all those who live in it. The city should embrace all its inhabitants as its citizens who have citizenship rights that include participation in urban planning and development and access to efficient public services, social protection and the opportunities of urban life.
- We individually and collectively build the city through our daily actions and our political, intellectual and economic engagements. We build economically productive communities with very little, if nonexistent, government support. We provide housing and essential services to ourselves. But when the communities we live in become valuable urban land, we are told to move out so the city can build on the debris of our homes and lives.
- We have a right to the city. This right is not merely a right of access to what property speculators and city planners define, but an active right to exercise urban citizenship. We imagine a more inclusive city based not

only upon the principles of human rights, but also upon the concept of the Right to the City.

"Urban Policies and the Right to the City: Rights, Responsibilities and Citizenship", a document produced in September 2008 at the request of UNESCO (by Alison Brown of the School of City and Regional Planning, Cardiff University and Annali Kristiansen of the Department for the Rule of Law, Danish Institute for Human Rights) underscores the Right to the City as having a real potential for enfranchisement and social inclusion and that many innovative tools and regional instruments have now been developed which, at least in part, translate the concept into practice. The Right to the City defines a series of legitimate claims to the conditions necessary for satisfying dignified and secure existence in cities by both individual citizens and social groups.

The concept of the Right to the City has been debated at five international meetings organized by UNESCO, UN-HABITAT and NGOs, in UNESCO Headquarters in Paris (2005, 2006), Barcelona (2005), Vancouver (2006) and Porto Alegre (2008). The meetings have identified the Right to the City "as a vehicle for urban change, in which all urban dwellers are urban citizens; it creates space in which citizens can define their needs but, in order to appropriate substantive citizenship, citizens must claim rights of participation, and allow others the same right."

Among the many initiatives to promote the Right to the City is a movement to develop a World Charter on the Right to the City, a theme that has been taken up in the World Social Forum movement.

The proposed Charter on the Right to the City defines the right as, "the equitable usufruct of cities within the principles of sustainability, democracy, equity and social justice", in which the right to the city is independent of all recognized rights, conceived as a whole open to incorporation of new rights." We resolve to take up the theme of the urban poor dwellers' Right to the City to define our struggle for a dignified and secure life in the city.

We further resolve to:

- Embark on a campaign at the national and regional level to change the notion about poor urban dwellers as an urban poor sector into a group of people who are citizens of the city that must no longer suffer social exclusion.
- Work together in movement building and strengthening, and building political and economic power in realizing humane homes, jobs and access to efficient public services.
- Take common actions towards building regional solidarity and pressing for social protection for poor urban dwellers.

THE GENDERED POLITICS OF ACCESS IN INDIA

The analysis in this chapter spans more than ten years (1994-2007). The chapter examines key feminist debates on political recruitment and in the context of India, three successful access routes that women have been able to make use of to enter the parliament in these ten years - support of family and kinship networks, participation in social and political movements and membership of political parties - are discussed and also one unsuccessful - quotas for women. Family networks continue to play an important role in women's access into parliamentary politics, while participation in social and political movements shows greater complexity.

Membership of political parties continues to be important as an access route for women but these organizations are also difficult terrains upon which to operate. While quotas can be a 'fast track' to increased representation in parliament, this route continues to be blocked to Indian women at present. So, although there have been some shifts in the patterns of access routes over the ten years covered by this research, family and political parties - to different extent - remain the key gateways to parliamentary politics.

WOMEN'S POLITICAL PARTICIPATION IN BANGLADESH

Political parties are the legitimate porters to elected office as they bear the responsibility of recruitment, selection and election of candidates. Political party's philosophy in regards to representation of women differs worldwide. Initiatives intended to ensure greater participation of women can take the form of reservation of quotas, target members or affirmative action measures. Reservation of quotas had been introduced at the local and central government level in Bangladesh with an intention to involve more women in the decision making process.

This chapter is an attempt to ascertain the role of political parties in the process of introduction of reservation of quotas for women. Emphasis will be given on the exploration of the role that political parties had played while the Local Government (Union Parishad) Second Amendment Act, 1997 was enacted through which reservation as well as provision of direct election for women was introduced. Along with ascertaining the role of political parties, efforts will also be given on the description of the present state of women's political participation in Bangladesh and to identify factors hindering the process of female political participation in Bangladesh.

EXPERIENTIAL REALM OF DALIT WOMEN IN BSP

This chapter seeks to understand the approaches of caste based political parties (who derive categories or certain identity politics) through accommodating gender in their respective parties. Gender, as a heterogeneous category, has serious linkages with factors like race, caste, religion, ethnicity, and so on. Hence, it is important to examine its different shades and its structures which determine gender in a deeper way in Indian society and its reflection in the realm of politics. The Chief Minister of U.P., Mayawati, in support of the Women's Reservation Bill, earlier argued that fifty percent reservation for women should be given.

In spite of constant struggle of women's organisation and women representative from various political parties WRB is agenda became unsuccessful. Moreover, one has to investigate some kind of alternative models such as gendering policy within the party system, especially, when the women themselves are the supremo within the party itself. This chapter tries to locate the position of Dalit women within Bahujan Samaj Party and further raise the question of the representation and accommodation of Dalit women within that party.

THE GENDERED TERRAIN OF PARTY POLITICS IN TAMIL NADU

Scholars of Tamil politics have convincingly argued that party political discourse in the southern Indian state of Tamil Nadu is highly gendered. More than a decade ago, a number of scholarly accounts showed how party politics was organized around the category of gender with significant ideological-discursive formations taking note of gendered categories. Within the DMK notions of women's chastity, purity, and honour were associated with the glory of the Tamil nation, and reified a woman's role as mother through the iconic figure of Tamilttay.

The other major regional party in state, the AIADMK, was profoundly influence by paternalistic leadership of the late MG Ramachandran, a film star-politician and former Chief Minister. We re-visit this literature after a decade and investigate the extent and manner in which political party organizations in Tamil Nadu are gendered institutions. This is particularly important given recent changes in Tamil party politics, with the rise of newer regionally based political parties entering politics at the state-level, as well as internal shifts in the two dominant parties.

GENDER AND THE CASE OF THE PATTALI MAKKAL KATCHI (PMK)

The issue of female sexuality became a major object of party political discourse in late 2005 following comments made by the popular film actress Kushboo. The theme is not new to Tamil Nadu with Periyar, the Self-Respect Movement and the Dravidar Kazhagam propagating the idea that marriage was a patriarchal institution.

However a number of political parties, including the DMK

earlier, have assumed the role of protectors of the honour of Tamils, and invoke the chastity of Tamil women as a symbol of that honour. The PMK instigated protests against Kushboo's comments bringing the issue of gender to salience once again in state politics. This chapter asks why the issue came to salience at this particular juncture and examines closely the gendered orientation of the party's strategy for mobilization.

THE EMERGENCE OF FEMALE PATRONS IN INDIA'S GLOBAL CITIES

This chapter looks at the performative and discursive ways by which female political subjects are produced out of formal and informal political and cultural processes framed by a political party that functions both within, and outside the state. I look at the party politics of women of a militant, political party in urban India, Shiv Sena (Shivaji's Army) to examine the emergence of what I refer to here as urban female "patrons" and "power-brokers."

The contest over Urbanisation that has been unleashed by transnational visions of urban space has opened up particularly significant spheres of influence for female party-workers at the local levels of Shiv Sena's functioning. I suggest that urban political power at the local and often informal levels of party activity is a continually negotiated process where constitutions of gendered personality become critical to the production of personal and political power.

Using data from extensive fieldwork conducted with women of the Shiv Sena party in the state of Maharashtra, I focus on specific cases of urban contest in the Indian cities of Mumbai and Pune to illustrate the emergence of female patrons and power-brokers and the performative constitution of gendered, urban political power.

THE POLITICAL FORMATIONS IN CONTEMPORARY HARYANA

Haryana, with geographical proximity to the national capital, is now increasingly seen as a crucial investment 'zone'.

But this state has a problematic socio-political formation which is grossly insensitive towards the weaker sections based on caste and gender. Here the social base and ideological compulsions of the dominant political parties are such that democratization of socio- economic structure is repeatedly obstacled.

There are numerous incidents of violence against women and Dalits, and on such gruesome issues the dominant political parties including Congress (I), INLD, BJP and others have taken a position that strengthens the oppressor and further intimidates the victim families. This attitude of the political parties necessitates an exposition of their ideological formation, which this chapter will do by foregrounding their limited notions and practices of social justice in Haryana.

This chapter will discuss specific cases of honor killings like Karora village in Kaithal district and that of Jhondi. The most vocal and consistent resistance is from AIDWA, ALL India Democratic Women Association as led by Jagmati Sangwan, a feminist activist in Haryana. This chapter is based on field work of interviews of the surviving victims, their families and AIDWA activists.

GENDER-SPECIFIC VIOLATIONS IN AFGHANISTAN

For the field of transitional justice, which seeks mechanisms and processes to reestablish peace and encourage accountability for past crimes and reconciliation within conflict-ridden communities, questions of violations that women suffer during conflicts are especially pertinent. Decoding the gendered nature of conflict and violations committed during such an event is complicated by the fact that women are often overlooked as actors and victims. Furthermore the crimes against women during such circumstances are seldom specific to outbreaks of war; the conflict merely accentuates discrimination and violations that women suffer during peace. In the context of post-conflict Afghanistan, the issue of past violations and gender is particularly vexing.

The U.S.-led military intervention in Afghanistan was legitimized in part with the rationale of "saving Afghan women" from the oppressive Taliban regime, and a language of empowerment of women and mainstreaming of gender has been integral in the state-building process in Afghanistan. At the formal level, Afghanistan has made some advances in the past eight years.

Yet close observers realized that removing the Taliban from power was not the end of the struggle for women's rights, or even the beginning. This was not a nation with a legacy of well-established, legally protected and socially accepted women's rights. The crippling legacy of decades of fighting has strained many of Afghanistan's social and political bonds. Little documented, the experience of Afghan women through the Soviet, civil and Taliban-era wars has been a particularly grueling one, and existing social biases and discrimination exacerbate the consequences of those conflicts. In addition, Afghanistan, especially outside its main urban centers, remains an intensely patriarchal society with complex tribal codes and customs circumscribing social interaction.

The relationship between women's and men's roles is marked by these codes and patterns. This four-part paper analyzes the relationship between transitional justice and gender in Afghanistan. First, it discusses transitional justice and gender in general, drawing on experiences from other post-conflict contexts. Second, it provides a brief overview of the three decades of conflict and the complex gender relations in Afghan society. Third, it discusses transitional justice and gender in the post-2001, state-building process in Afghanistan. And last it concludes with recommendations. Research for this chapter began in January 2007 and lasted through March 2008.

The International Center for Transitional Justice (ICTJ) also conducted training on documenting gender-specific violations in Kabul for the Afghan Independent Human Rights Commission (AIHRC) and United Nations Development Fund for Women (UNIFEM) in December 2007.

GENDER AND TRANSITIONS

Gender and Transitional Justice In recent decades there has been an increased focus on transitional justice and the rule of law in both conflict and post-conflict societies, with transitional justice strategies seen as a necessary step in promoting justice for past abuses and building national unity and reconciliation. Justice, peace and democracy should not be seen as mutually exclusive goals but rather as mutually reinforcing imperatives. Advancing all of these goals in fragile, post-conflict settings requires strategic planning, careful integration and sensible sequencing of events. The challenges of dealing with post-conflict environments require an approach that balances a variety of goals, including the pursuit of accountability, truth and reparation; the preservation of peace; and the building of genuine democracy and the rule of law.

Any transitional justice approach should include both judicial and non-judicial mechanisms and should seek to encompass broadly the various dimensions of justice that can heal wounds and contribute to social reconstruction based on a fundamental belief in universal human rights. While men's experiences of conflict have been well documented, women's experiences have often been overlooked. Until very recently many truth commission mandates, criminal justice approaches, judicial opinions, policy proposals for reparations and other transitional justice mechanisms have paid little or no attention to the suffering of women.

Some progress has been made in the following areas: the use of thematic gender hearings in truth commissions; ensuring that data collected is disaggregated on the basis of gender; new jurisprudence on gendered crimes at an international level; and a greater focus on addressing specific gender crimes in reparations programmes. Women have participated in transitional justice processes as victims and survivors of conflict, as well as witnesses, combatants, perpetrators and transitional justice activists. As victims and survivors, they are perceived traditionally as secondary victims or survivors of war. In reality, they are usually the primary victims.

During conflicts, the physical crimes against women include death, sexual violence and harm to their reproductive systems through forced pregnancy and sterilization. The long-term consequences of conflict include economic hardship, health violations, fewer legal rights and questions of access to land. The increased focus on gender and on women's experiences advance the rights of women and to advance gender justice by considering some pressing issues:

- Communities often stigmatize female ex-combatants both as part of conflict and for stepping out of traditional gender roles by taking up arms;
- Reintegration too often focuses on economic and social reintegration, and fails to address the psychological, social and medical needs of women;
- As principal caregivers in most societies especially where medical and other infrastructures have collapsed, women are often responsible for the reintegration of their kin, many of whom are injured and traumatized. Transitional justice measures need to examine the roles of women as agents of reintegration;
- Women and girls play multiple roles in combat that are not always recognized, from cooks and porters to guards and fighters.

Seventy-two percent of the girls within the Lord's Resistance Army operating in Northern Uganda received weapons and military training. As a sign of their willingness to "talk peace," 1,000 of the LRA boys were released; only 15 girls were let go because they were seen as less valuable.

PROSECUTIONS

Pursuing judicial accountability for human rights violations, either through domestic or international bodies, has been one avenue for establishing responsibility for and broadening awareness of massive and systematic crimes against women. Sexual violence during times of war and social upheaval has been rampant. Until recently, rape was not treated as a war crime against women or as the *actus reus* for genocide but rather as a crime against dignity and honor. This has changed in the last decade as the jurisprudence of the international tribunals have recognized that rape and other forms of sexual violence can constitute genocide, torture and other inhuman acts.

The prosecutor's office in the International Criminal Tribunal for Yugoslavia committed substantial resources to the question of gender and the prosecution of rape and sexual violence. This included appointing a legal advisor for gender-related crimes and developing special procedural protections, both in relation to evidentiary rules for prosecuting gender crimes and affording protective measures to safeguard the physical and mental wellbeing of victims and witnesses. The work of the ad hoc tribunals certainly influenced the mandate of the International Criminal Court. That court explicitly recognizes rape, sexual slavery, enforced prostitution, forced pregnancy, gender-based persecution, enforced sterilization and sexual violence as war crimes and crimes against humanity.

Despite the advances made by the ad hoc tribunals in prosecuting rape and sexual violence, many women say such changes have been more symbolic in nature because there has been very little follow-up in terms of prosecutions. In support of this critique, many scholars and activists argue that the rules of relevance, the establishment of culpability, the efficiency of judicial resources, and the protection of the due process rights of defendants influence against the right of victims and witnesses to tell their stories. They argue that this kind of truth-telling is not within the jurisdiction of formal legal forums and that the translation of human suffering into a vocabulary and form that is acceptable and appropriate to a judicial proceeding can be a dehumanizing experience for victims of sexual violence.

The reduction of gender to simply sexual violence against women is to ignore the gendered dimensions of conflict. These criticisms of the work of the ad hoc tribunals are not intended to suggest that prosecutions should be abandoned. Instead, our intent is to raise awareness of the complexity of understanding the gendered dimensions of conflict and the need to ensure that we critically explore our methodology so that in future applications we can do better. In this regard the Special Court of Sierra Leone has been in the unique position of operating currently with the country's truth and reconciliation commission.

The prosecutor made sexual violence one of the court's priorities and also identified in the indictments against the Revolutionary United Front (RUF) and the Armed Forces Revolutionary Council (AFRC) the crime of "forced marriage" as an inhuman act and crime against humanity under the courts statute.

TRUTH COMMISSIONS

The work and reports of truth commissions have become valuable tools in dealing with gender and violence against women. Generally established as official state bodies that investigate and report on human rights abuses, truth commissions also seek to make recommendations to remedy and prevent similar crimes in the future. In the past, however, the mandates of most truth commissions have not explicitly addressed the question of gender-specific crimes. In South Africa, intense lobbying from activists ensured that gender and the examination of the experience of women during the conflict was placed on the truth commission's agenda. As a result, the commission held special hearings for women and began to explore how the era of apartheid impacted women.

Part of the mandate of Sierra Leone's truth commission was to focus on the experiences of women and in particular, the sexual violence that occurred in the conflict period. However the commission went further and highlighted the structural injustices that women had experienced as a result of gender inequalities in Sierra Leone in the period before, during and after the conflict. The extensive findings provided an account of how social, legal, political and cultural forces conspired to render women more vulnerable during the conflict. The commission's recommendations, if implemented, should strengthen the position of women in Sierra Leonean society and make them less vulnerable to future victimization. The Liberian truth commission's mandate also requires that the commission explore gender and the experiences of women.

REPARATIONS

Women have been known to play crucial roles during periods of violence and its aftermath in searching for victims or their remains, trying to sustain and reconstitute families and communities and carrying on the tasks of unveiling the past and demanding justice. Yet reparations programmes to help victims of human rights violations have not focused on the forms of victimization that women are more commonly subject to, nor are the programmes designed with an explicit gender dimension in mind. This gap is noticeable in view of the different reparations programmes that have been implemented around the world in transitional democracies including those in South Africa, Germany, Chile, Brazil and Argentina.

Reparations refer to state-sponsored initiatives designed to compensate victims for the material and moral damages of past abuse. They typically distribute a mix of material and symbolic benefits to victims, which may include money and official apologies. The trend now has been an incipient trend to reverse the marginalization of victims in the discussions and practice of reparations. Sexual violence against women during times of conflict and authoritarianism is increasingly being discussed in relation to prosecutorial mechanisms and to reparations. There is a growing sense that including sexual violence among the violations deserving reparations is not the only issue; concerns with gender justice should somehow be "mainstreamed" in the discussions and design of reparations.

Still, there is little general understanding of what this may require. The truth commissions in Sierra Leone, Timor-Leste and Morocco have been among the few to address the specific nature of gender in conflicts through their respective reparations programmes and recommendations in their final reports. This is an area that needs more attention from all transitional justice structures. Ultimately any transitional justice process adopted should aim to empower women and reverse a discriminatory environment. This requires a broader focus on systemic violations than is currently the norm. It also requires that those involved go beyond established dogmas regarding gender, justice and transition, and initiate innovative measures and practices to ensure inclusion.

Furthermore, successful transitional justice priorities and approaches should ensure accountability for the victimized communities through local ownership supported by transnational solidarity. Any transitional justice approach adopted should pay attention to historical legacies and political contexts, taking into account that there are no universal solutions, only a series of past experiences and identified lessons that should be incorporated into the specific context of each transitioning society.

CONFLICT AND GENDER IN AFGHANISTAN

Afghanistan's Legacy of Conflict and War "Every conceivable human rights violation is occurring in Afghanistan, and on an enormous scale." These words from a report in 1984 could be said of the country's plight during the last three decades. The Afghan-Soviet war triggered a relentless cycle of violence and devastation that continued long after the last Soviet troops withdrew. Observers and analysts frequently mention of Afghanistan's "three eras of conflict"- the Soviet war, the civil war and the war with the Taliban. This unintentionally creates an impression of consistency and similarities between the different phases of conflict, hiding differences in types and magnitude of violations. The immediate and long-term impact of the Afghan-Soviet war laid the groundwork for much of Afghanistan's later and ongoing conflict. The massive violations committed during this period remain largely undocumented.

The few existing reports reveal a tragic picture of a civilian population that endured the excesses of a brutal war and occupation, including indiscriminate attacks, bombings and killings, and whose homes, land and property was destroyed or looted. Persecution on political and religious grounds was ubiquitous. Soviet officials and the Soviet-backed Afghan government routinely imprisoned people for political reasons, enforced disappearance torture, and summary executions were systematic practices. Afghanistan's intelligentsia and professional class were destroyed through imprisonment, execution or exile. Women were targeted for abduction, rape and other sexual violations, either randomly or during torture; they were often attacked and killed with their children because the men in many communities had to abandon their homes either to fight or avoid capture and execution.

Villages and roads, once razed, were scattered with mines. Between one to two million Afghans died and another five to six million were displaced. The Soviet defeat and withdrawal gave Afghanistan only a short respite. Then civil war broke out. The civilian population in Kabul, which had been spared the worst excesses of the previous war, was now targeted by infighting among former *mujahidin* factions who turned their guns upon each other. By this time, the Cold War was over; hence Afghanistan retreated in the Western conscience and consciousness. As a result, most reporting of human rights violations in the course of the four-year civil war came after 2001, when interest in Afghanistan was rekindled after the fall of the Taliban. Tens of thousands of civilians died in indiscriminate bombings, rocket fire, executions and massacres.

Torture was used often to coerce and terrorize the population, and rape became a systematic violation during the civil war. The Uttar anarchy from 1992 to 1996 made even the Taliban a welcome force for stability, but not for long. A Pakistani-backed movement, the Taliban drew much support from Afghan refugee camps along the Afghan-Pakistani border and in *mudarris* (religious grammar schools). In the heavily factionalized and fragmented country, Taliban leaders demonstrated they could impose order, first taking control of Qandahar in the south and eventually proceeding to Kabul. Persistent fighting between the Taliban and the loosely grouped Northern Alliance resulted in numerous massacres of civilians throughout the country from 1996 to 2001.

Mass arrests, torture and extrajudicial executions were also common tactics, both among Taliban and Northern Alliance forces. In some areas, the Taliban adopted a scorched-earth policy, killing civilians, razing villages, looting property, and destroying land and crops. The Taliban pursued stringent policies toward women by restricting freedom of movement, prohibiting them from attending schools or getting jobs, and enforcing mandatory veiling through its Ministry of the Prevention of Vice and the Promotion of Virtue.

TRADITION, RELIGION AND PATRIARCHY

The different phases of the conflict and the ideologies of regimes in power have contributed to the suffering of Afghan women, as they have been the direct and indirect victims of all fighting in the country. However, describing the situation for women in Afghanistan through the lens of past and present conflict runs the risk of hiding the production of unequal gender relations through the complex web of conflict, religion, custom and poverty. Afghan society remains largely pre-industrial, agrarian and impoverished. The Afghan-Soviet war destroyed the modest economic gains of the 1950s and 1960s, and unrelenting conflict from the 1980s onward continues to impede development. The link between industrial development, Urbanisation and gender dynamics is significant, as the demand for labor in industrial societies has often helped women shift from the private to the public sphere.

The earliest attempts to modernize Afghan society came in the early 20th century during the reign of King Amanullah, who, after Afghanistan's independence in 1919, sought sweeping reforms in constitutional law, trade and education. His equally ambitious efforts to restructure Afghanistan's social relations through legal reform and more controversially, banning public veiling - were received much less enthusiastically. After Amanullah abdicated in 1929, most of his reforms were abandoned. Several decades later in the 1970s,

Communist governments put forward similar sweeping reforms, particularly in the area of education, in order to uproot what they considered to be backward traditional and religious norms and practices within Afghan society.

This rise to power of the secular but brutal regime and its subsequent collapse drew a backlash from the most conservative elements of Afghan society. Savage infighting between former mujahidin who had fought Russia in the 1980s created more violence and chaos throughout the country, until the Taliban movement managed to push back and hold most other paramilitary groups to the north of the country. The Taliban regime proved particularly vicious to women, non-Pashtuns and urban dwellers that tended to disagree with the rigid tribal and religious customs the Taliban made law. In urban centers such as Kabul (the capital) women were barred from working and girls' schools throughout the country were shut down.

Less comfortable for observers to acknowledge, perhaps, is that the Taliban's vision for social order was not entirely alien to large segments of Afghan society. Many of the government's laws, particularly with respect to women, were an extension of the complex tribal codes and social customs already in effect in the Pashtun south. Castigating the Taliban as the primary offenders of women's rights in Afghanistan is unhelpful and misleading, as it fails to confront the deeper social forces that produce and reinforce patriarchal norms that predate the Taliban movement. Religion and custom define men's attitudes toward women in Afghan society, though with differing degrees of significance. In addition, socioeconomic class is a strong determinant of gender relations. Especially since the attacks on the United States in September 2001, perceived misogyny within Islam is often used to explain "the woman question."

In the Afghan context and on the face of it, the argument seems legitimate; literalist interpretations of religion are used to enforce rules and regulate social interactions, and to give the authority of men over women moral credibility. Certainly during Taliban rule, the sentences for "moral" and ordinary crimes often manifesting in brutal and highly visible ways such as public stoning for adultery or amputation of limbs for theft came from the harshest readings possible of sharia (Islamic law). Then and now, however, the Islamic legal system in Afghanistan reveals serious flaws, gaps in jurisprudential understanding, and a tenuous grasp of the vast, cumbersome body of law that constitutes sharia.

Lack of access to basic and higher education, even for religious scholars or judges, has ensured the disintegration of most formal Islamic learning and has impoverished the debate over religious and legal issues in Afghanistan. The understanding of Islam and especially Islamic jurisprudence has also become intimately intertwined with the different customary frameworks of Afghanistan. In Afghanistan, women activists argue that gender dynamics are better examined through prisms of custom and tradition than religion. Afghanistan remains poor and rural, with most tribes, communities and villages observing the same patterns of daily life and interaction as they have for centuries, the upheavals of war notwithstanding.

An evocative saying captures the Afghan attitude toward girls and young women: "Why tend flowers meant for someone else's garden?" In practice, this has meant that girls, once married, are not able to contribute to sustaining her parents' family. Since girls are not viewed as able to generate income even when unmarried, they are seen as economic burdens to be shifted to husbands as early as possible. Under these conditions, child marriages are practiced widely, particularly as poorer families can get sizeable dowries for their daughters. Criminalization of child marriage has had little impact, in part because neither births nor marriages are routinely registered. Viewing young girls as economic burdens (and also as financial leverage) effectively means they are ultimately no more than saleable, tradable property. Indeed, young and single women are frequently used to settle internecine conflict between families or tribes in a practice known as *baad* (literally, to trade).

Blood disputes, financial agreements, debts and almost any other kind of exchange can be transacted with women as currency. Because girls and women frequently have no means of securing financial independence, marriage is the safest bid for a stable future, though by no means a guarantee of it. Prioritizing male children within families, coupled with early marriages, high maternal mortality rates, and low life expectancy, limited access to education and ongoing poverty ensures that from one generation to the next, women are not able improve their quality of life. Intertwined with the view of women as passive objects rather than as individuals is the concept of honor and dignity. The patriarchal frameworks in Afghanistan paradoxically designate women (rather than men themselves) as the vessels of familial and communal honour.

Gender segregation (which predates the Taliban) is a direct consequence of the need to protect women's honor from other men. Notions of honor, however, do not exist for their own sake; again, they are intimately tied to a girl's economic value. Girls who are not virgins, for example, are devalued and not eligible for marriage, even if they were victims of rape. Girls and women who flee their homes because they are subject to violence or domestic abuse are seen as equally tainted; no one can answer for a girl's honor if she was unsupervised outside the reach of her male family members. Indeed, women are frequently imprisoned for leaving their homes, even though it is not actually a crime. In Afghanistan's main urban centers, some of the social constraints and norms that prevail in the provinces are less obvious.

Women and girls work, attend schools and universities, and are permitted more freedom of movement. However, educated women remain open to varying levels of harassment and violence throughout the country, with numerous cases of female politicians, civil servants, activists and academics facing challenges within their professional and private lives. In previous decades, the contrast between urban and rural areas has been equally marked with respect to women's roles, and this divide remains entrenched. Socioeconomics played a critical role: in the 1960s and 1970s; families who were significantly richer or politically connected also espoused much freer social behavior to a degree unprecedented in Afghanistan.

Access to education is also key issue because this usually provides women with greater opportunities to be employed and self-sufficient. As a rule, industrial and urban centers provide these prospects. In examining the link between gender and development, consider some of the indicators for Afghanistan with respect to women. Afghan women have a life expectancy of 44 years. They face one of the highest maternal mortality rates in the world. Between 90 and 95 percent of all Afghan women are illiterate. Afghanistan's Gender Development Index is the third lowest in the world. Although primary school enrollment increased post-2001, the country's school enrollment rates are among the lowest globally, with half the number of girls enrolled as boys; in the southern provinces, only 15 percent of schoolchildren are female.

TRANSITIONAL JUSTICE AND GENDER

The international military intervention in Afghanistan in 2001 and the following democratization process gave the country an opportunity to address its violent past and to break with gender-based discrimination and abuse. While the majority of Afghans have welcomed the end of the Taliban regime, the transition in 2001 fell short of being a fresh start for the Afghan people. Security, poverty and lack of economic development remain major concerns for most Afghans. Compromised governance, rule of law and security-sector reforms have eroded support for President Hamid Karzai's government and for the international presence in Afghanistan.

The Bonn Agreement, the roadmap for the first five years of the state-building process, did not include a framework for transitional justice. However, it established the AIHRC that was later mandated to address past crimes. In a nationwide survey the AIHRC conducted in 2004, Afghans voiced overwhelming support for a comprehensive political accountability process to prosecute people widely suspected of mass human rights abuses and crimes against humanity over the past 30 years. Encompassing views and findings from 4,000 interviews with people from every province, the report conveys a strong demand for accountability for the crimes of each previous regime.

Though men and women were included in focus groups and interviews, and notable differences in responses were found between the sexes, the interviews and findings do not contain specific sections that address gender-related crimes or the views of the women who responded. In December 2005, the Afghan government signed the Action Plan for Peace, Reconciliation and Justice (hereafter the Action Plan). This is structured around five key action points, the most contentious of which calls for the establishment of "effective and reasonable accountability mechanisms" to end and prevent further impunity by ensuring war criminals and perpetrators of human rights abuses do not get amnesty. While the plan makes passing reference to the question of gender-based violations, it has made little substantive headway in addressing the fundamental social and political imbalances that have permitted abuses against women.

The Action Plan received a boost in January 2006 when the Afghan government and the international community made its implementation a condition of the Afghanistan Compact and the ensuing Afghan National Development Strategy (ANDS); this incorporated the plan into one of its three central pillars, that of Governance, Rule of Law, and Human Rights, and aims for its completion by the end of 2008. Corruption control and gender equality are cross-sector issues within this ANDS pillar, but corruption remains a central concern to the donor community and governance specialists. Documentation of violations against women in Afghanistan from the various periods of conflict exists from various sources. Most recently, the AIHRC is conducting a human rights mapping exercise that aims to produce a comprehensive overview of the last three eras of conflict in

Afghanistan and constitutes a central pillar within the transitional justice process.

Other efforts to document human rights violations include an unpublished conflict mapping report from the Office of the High Commissioner for Human Rights. Organizations such as the *Afghanistan Justice Project, Amnesty International, Human Rights Watch and the Human Rights Research and Advocacy Consortium* have also tried to shed light on violations against women from a factual perspective rather than one incorporating a gendered analysis. The transitional justice process in Afghanistan now runs the risk of total political marginalization. Officials within the Afghan government and international community as well as civil society organizations agree that the momentum and political will needed to implement the Action Plan no longer exist. In March 2007, the Afghan parliament passed a law extending amnesty to all armed groups and leaders who have operated in the country over the last 25 years.

The implementation of this law could consolidate the culture of impunity that pervades the highest level of Afghanistan's government. Indeed, in the months following, many individuals and groups have found themselves at a loss as to how they could take concrete action within the transitional justice process. In an environment where transitional justice remains highly politicized and little official will exists, the burden for action has been taken up by extremely nascent and vulnerable civil society organizations.

MAINSTREAMING OF GENDER AND WOMEN'S RIGHTS

The rights of Afghan women served as the cause célèbre of many organizations during Taliban rule, rising to a fever pitch after the U.S.-led invasion in 2001. Afghan women and the international public, the thinking went, needed protection from radical Islamic fundamentalism; overthrowing the Taliban would serve both purposes. The years between the Taliban's ascent to and fall from power saw a veritable frenzy of literature, academic writing and films about the plight of

Afghan women. In 2005 the United Nations Special Rapporteur (UNSR) on *Violence Against Women*, Yakin Ertük, conducted a mission to Afghanistan.

Her report concluded that four major dynamics are at the root of the "dramatic and severe violence" Afghan women face: Afghanistan's patriarchal social order, the erosion of protective social mechanisms, the absence of rule of law and poverty and insecurity. The report highlighted a series of ongoing, widespread violations such as domestic violence, rape, trafficking, abduction, forced marriage, selling or trading girls to settle debts, "honor killings" and lack of access to education, health services and due process. Since 2001, the Afghan government has taken several steps at the highest levels to promote the rights of women.

Constitutional reform, the creation of ministry to deal with women's issues, and attempts to mainstream gender into the country's development strategies are the Karzai administration's most high-profile endeavors. The creation of the Ministry of Women's Affairs (MoWA) was an acknowledgment that gender issues in Afghanistan needed attention and oversight at the highest levels. As the central policymaking unit that would uphold women's rights and mainstream women's involvement in every aspect of the national and provincial governments, the ministry faces crippling difficulties beyond the resource and capacity constraints that hamstring all Afghan government agencies. As one official said, a silent political resistance surrounds every issue as well as any organisation that seeks to work on any aspect of gender issues; the resistance becomes vocal and violent when members of parliament call for MoWA to be closed, or a provincial representative of the ministry is gunned down.

Frequent changes in the ministry's leadership (four ministers in the past five years) undermine the agency's work and institutional memory. MoWA is not yet able to fulfill its role as the main policy driver on women's issues and has instead devolved into a secondary role, providing a range of resources and support services to women that, while badly needed, distort the ministry's ability to build its expertise and consolidate its function as a government body that keeps women's issues at the top of the policy agenda. So, while the intentions behind creating the ministry were good, MoWA has had the unintended effect of allowing policymakers to marginalize gender as being the problem of just one government office, rather than an issue that needs to be integrated into all departments.

The National Action Plan for the Women of Afghanistan (NAPWA) - developed under MoWA leadership - is included as a benchmark in ANDS. Gender mainstreaming has its own component within ANDS' Governance, Rule of Law, and Human Rights pillar and is moreover a theme throughout the entire strategy. However, the gap between ANDS' objectives and current progress in the area of gender rights is staggering. The Joint Consultation and Monitoring Board (JCMB), the high-level panel charged with overseeing the implementation of ANDS, has consistently neglected the activities and benchmarks within the gender mainstreaming agenda. None of recent quarterly JCMB meetings have discussed or inquired about NAPWA's progress.

Article 22 of the Afghan Constitution declares: "Any kind of discrimination and privilege between the citizens of Afghanistan are prohibited. The citizens of Afghanistan - whether man or woman have equal rights and duties before the law." Article 44 states that: "The state shall devise and implement effective programmes for balancing and promoting of education for women, improving of education of nomads and elimination of illiteracy in the country." Other clauses on the National Assembly establish quotas for female representation in the upper and lower houses of the legislature. Limited efforts have been made to put the values and rights of the Constitution into practice.

For example, the inclusion of the equal rights clause in the Afghan Constitution in 2004 was not pre-dated or followed by a comprehensive review to identify whether the laws existing in Afghanistan conform to the equal rights guarantee.

The domestic legal framework does not provide adequate protection for women and girls from gender-based crimes. Rape is not a codified offense under Afghan law, and rape victims are often prosecuted under the adultery provisions of the Penal Code of 1976. Article 77 of the Civil Laws allows marriages to be contracted without the woman's consent, and Article 517 of the Penal Code criminalizes the practice of "giving" females for marriage or *baad* only when the party is a widow or at least 18 years old.

The judicial system needs systematic rebuilding at every level. Strategies and plans have been put forward for its reform, yet as a whole, the reform of the justice sector lags behind. The confusion, inefficiency and corruption of the formal justice systems mean that the majority of Afghans turn to it as a last resort; most cases, whether civil or criminal, are considered and settled within customary tribal mechanisms. At the risk of simplification, it may be fair to say that Afghan police fail to recognize crimes against women, or detain women for activities that are not crimes at all (as mentioned, when women flee their homes, they are often arrested even though no such crime exists in any of Afghanistan's legal codes). ICTJ has conducted assessments on the complementary, but separate issue of developments and difficulties in the area of women's rights.

It also has examined the links between the lack of access of justice for women and the past and present impunity for government officials that continue to erode security, stability and the rule of law. Women continue to face the same patterns and sorts of abuse as in previous decades; longstanding and deeply prejudiced cultural mores, conflation of religious and tribal practices, an almost nonexistent legal system, and law enforcement officials who give violations of women's rights short shrift doubly exacerbate the situation. The constant refrain from Afghans is that the processes to institute and maintain the rule of law in the provinces are faltering.

The population's confidence in the government to deliver basic necessities and ensure a modicum of stability and access to justice is slipping dangerously, in part because of a sense that the current government cares neither for redressing abuses of the past nor for preventing abuses of the present. Considerations of gender and women's experiences of conflict have not been a dominant thread in the nascent transitional justice process in Afghanistan. Although other initiatives have sought to focus equally on women and men, women's experiences of the conflict remain marginalized. At the same time, gender policies designed and implemented by the Afghan government and its international partners tend to limit their analyses of legacies of the past, and in doing so overlook its significance in their plans for the future.

As a result, there is limited understanding of how the manifold legacies of the past have affected the lives of Afghan women and gender relations in Afghanistan today. No monolithic classification of women exists in Afghanistan. Women's experiences differ depending on geography, ethnicity and social class. However, analyzing gender relations in Afghanistan demands multiple layers of knowledge, in particular about the ways in which the legacies of conflict, poverty and illiteracy interact and affect the lives of families and communities. Understanding gender in Afghanistan requires grasping the continuum of violations and deprivations that shape women's lives. This area of inquiry is not well understood because most data and information is anecdotal, incomplete or simply nonexistent. For example, what is the situation of women forced into marriage during previous conflict?

What is the situation of their children? How do women who have experienced sexual violence during the conflict cope? How do their families and communities address these issues? This briefing does not address gender and transitional justice in Afghanistan at a detailed level; it is an overview of challenges and considerations. ICTJ puts forward the following recommendations to deepen the understandings of the interplay between considerations of gender and past and ongoing violations:

1. Furthering research: Through our research, we have realized that very limited resources and information

currently exist on gender and transitional justice in Afghanistan. One major example of an unexamined issue (but by no means the only one) is that of researching and distinguishing between those gender-based violations that stem directly from conflict and violations that occur during peacetime or as indirect products of conflict. Another major analytical weakness is the failure of many to consider violations against women within the continuum of conflict and against the background of poverty, illiteracy and entrenched patriarchal systems. A critical need remains for further research that takes into account women's experiences of conflict and of how the country's broader experience with conflict continues to affect gender relations in Afghanistan.

2. Analyzing and drawing upon comparative experiences: Afghanistan can learn from the experiences of other countries where gender considerations have been taken into account when addressing legacies of the past. As described, there has been a learning curve in other countries with respect to including women's experiences and gender dimensions in documentation, victims' advocacy and in more formal transitional justice mechanisms, such as truth commissions. It is vital to relate and contextualize these experiences in Afghanistan.
3. Pursuing documentation: As certain elements of this chapter have suggested, the transitional justice process in Afghanistan must pay special attention to the country's women, particularly in documentation, research and truth-seeking efforts, an endeavor that has been minimal to date. Though anecdotal data suggests the scale and nature of violations that women face, very little qualitative or quantitative research or trend analysis exists on past violence against women, whether domestic violence or war crimes. In this vacuum, information collected on gender-based violence becomes more significant in establishing a historical record of women's experiences. Documentation then forms a critical element of the transitional justice process for Afghanistan. Though the

country remains in a state of conflict, an immediate, urgent need exists to document widely and accurately the testimonies and accounts of what the population has witnessed in the last three decades of war.

4. Encouraging the growth and capacity of victims' groups: In the absence of formal or state-led transitional justice processes, civil society has frequently played a central role in fostering and enriching discussions of accountability and reconciliation within society at large and advocating for the rights of the survivors of conflict. Nascent organizations in Afghanistan are attempting to do the same and often find themselves in a difficult position when dealing with questions of gender. Many human rights or victims' organizations find themselves at a loss when addressing gender-based violations, because the definition of victimization is unclear (are women victimized by conflict or by broader socioeconomic conditions?), the stigma of being the victim of sexual violations (whether female or male) is so large, and so few support services exist.

4

Gender as Destiny

In 2001, Afghanistan embarked upon a new beginning with the overthrow of the Taliban regime, recognizing anew the contribution of the female half of its society. After years of minimal involvement of women in public life, the Bonn Agreement called for specific attention to the role of women and established a dedicated government structure for this purpose, the Ministry of Women's Affairs.

The core strategy for women's advancement is defined as 'gender progress towards gender equality is a critical issue for us. .....First we will adopt measures to restore those rights to our women and girls that they were denied because of the segregationist policies of the Taliban and the threat to their personal security during periods of conflict. To support this, we will need to create women's specific opportunities that will allow them to catch up with men and boys. Particular concerns are the re-instatement of women in employment and income-earning opportunities, up-grading women's professional knowledge which has fallen out of date because of their years of exclusion, and enhancing their management skills and familiarity with modern technologies in the work place. These will call for specific programmes directed to enhancing the capabilities of our girls and women'.

After two decades of conflict, destruction and massive displacement of its population, Afghanistan is faced with unprecedented challenges and the daunting task of building institutions and capacity to forge a pathway to progress, outlined in the strategic document *Securing Afghanistan's Future* in March 2004. The successful conduct of the Constitutional *Loya Jirga* in December 2003 and the Presidential Election in October 2004 constituted important milestones in this regard.

Despite Constitutional gender equality before the law since 1964, the legal framework guiding Afghan women's lives consists of a mixture of customary law, Islamic Law and traditions, all of which stress the complementarities of male and female roles more than their equality. Within this larger framework, there are considerable regional differences in the position of women and even more, between rural and urban areas and between educated and non-educated groups in society.

PROCESS OF THE COUNTRY GENDER ASSESSMENT

In support of the government's efforts and policies, the World Bank has prepared this Country Gender Assessment to identify critical areas in which gender-responsive actions are likely to enhance growth, poverty reduction and human well-being. The extent of gender discrimination in Afghanistan is pervasive, and the present report focuses on a few key sectors deemed particularly important for both short and long-term reconstruction. Gender gaps in Afghanistan are widespread in health, in education, in economic opportunities and in power and political voice. While women and girls bear the direct cost of these inequalities, and the negative effects are felt throughout the society.

The Country Gender Assessment makes the case that improvements in women's situation are essential for the reconstruction of the country - and that sizable investments in this regard will yield large benefits. Political and social turmoil allowed little research and national level data collection in the past few decades, and few empirical analyses have been conducted, leading to a gap in systematic knowledge about gender relations beyond anecdotal evidence.

As a result, the approach chosen here has been to assemble a situational report covering the main issues in key sectors of gender inequality such as health, education, agriculture, employment and legal rights.

The objective of this Assessment is to identify the key issues relating to gender mainstreaming in the Afghan context, notably to women's involvement in the development process both as beneficiaries and contributors. In order to achieve this objective, the approach chosen has been on the one hand to document the unequal access to services, resources and economic opportunities and the major obstacles to achieving equity, and on the other hand to document women's significant but largely ignored, contribution to the household and national economy, and the constraints to expanding women's economic role.

This documentation of the equity deficits for women in various sectors is put in a wider gender perspective in the chapter on women's legal position and voice inside and outside the household, where some of the most deep-rooted factors behind the present gender inequity can be identified in the form of women's highly unequal legal position and almost complete lack of voice at all levels of society. As part of the process of formulating the Country Gender Assessment, a workshop was held in Kabul in September 2004, to which a wide range of international and national agencies active in the various sectors covered by this report were invited.

The goal was to gather information about good practices and lessons learned and to benefit from the insight gained by various agencies that have been working in Afghanistan in some cases for more than two decades and whose expertise too rarely is drawn upon outside their own programmes. Almost three quarters of the participants were Afghans, which also reflects the considerable local competence which has been built up over the years.

THE GENDER CONTEXT

In Afghanistan, the role of women and their position in the society are inextricably interlinked with the national destiny. Women are symbols of family honor but also carry the burden of embodying the national honor and aspirations of the country. Gender has thus been one of the most politicized issues in Afghanistan over the past 100 years, where many reform attempts rightly or wrongly have been condemned by opponents as un-Islamic and a challenge to the sanctity of the faith and family. Notions of honor and shame underpinning cultural norms and practices emphasize female modesty and purity and define men as breadwinners and the protectors of the family.

In 1929, the reformist king Amanullah's government fell soon after he tried to impose social reforms, including the abolition of *purdah* (separation and veiling of women) and establishment of coeducation. It took another 30 years before Mohammad Daoud, the then Prime Minister, in 1959, officially encouraged women to give up *purdah* and challenged the view that full veiling was a religious obligation. In the late 1970s, the leaders of the Communist (PDPA) regime which took power in 1978 pushed new reforms including elimination of the "bride-price" and forced adult education for women, which caused much of the rhetoric of the opposition to the PDPA-regime and Soviet occupation, to be formulated as a *"jihad"* and as protecting women from communist forces bent on destroying their purity and Islamic values.

Men's primary role thus became as Defenders of the Faith (*mujahedin*) and Protectors of the Honor of the Nation and the Family. In the 1990s, women's rights in Afghanistan remained a divisive issue. When the PDPA regime finally collapsed in 1992, and a coalition of *mujahedin* parties was installed in Kabul, decrees were announced instructing women to observe *hijab* i.e. covering of the head, arms, and legs. Local commanders in other cities announced similar decrees.

During the conflict and civil war in the 1980s and 1990s, particularly between 1992 and 1995, armed factions turned the traditional norms of honor and shame into weapons of war, engaging in rape and sexual assault against women of opposing groups as an ultimate means of dishonoring entire communities and reducing people's capacities to resist military advances. In response, concerns about women's security led to the imposition of ever stricter interpretations of what constitutes socially acceptable behavior, supported by the most conservative reading of the Holy Scriptures.

This development culminated under the Taliban regime whose views on gender denied women any role outside the immediate family and resulted in policies violating the very honor and sanctity of the family which they claimed to defend and relegated gender discourse to the realm of religious interpretations. The definition of gender roles is so central in Afghan society and culture, that any perceived or planned changes require consultations not only with the household but also with the larger community. Men and women to a large extent share the same cultural ethos and values, including their conception of gender roles, and they seek to validate these within their communities.

Years of turmoil have furthermore left communities to their own devices, strengthening the inherent distrust of external authorities and increased reliance upon conservative values. The remarkable social cohesion, which has brought the Afghan population through the years of turmoil with fewer scars than could be expected, also includes strict social norms and control of conformity with these norms. Hence any perceived attempt of inducing change requires solid consultation with and consent among the affected communities. Today, the estimated population of Afghanistan is around 24 million and it has a per capita GDP close to US$315 (including the opium economy), which is one of the lowest in the world.

Moreover, the country's social indicators are among the worst in the world, and with large gender gaps. Afghanistan has some of the worst health, educational and economic indicators in the world. Two decades of internecine warfare have led not only to a breakdown of infrastructure and services, but also have destroyed the livelihood of the people and contributed to the downward trend of women's rights.

By the end of 2001 government services, including health care and education, had stopped functioning, resulting in significant negative impacts particularly on women and children.

According to the National Human Development Report (2004) Afghanistan ranks 173rd out of 178 countries in the UN's Human Development Index and when in terms of its Gender Development Index only Niger and Burkina Faso are placed lower. However, parallel with the gradual development of democratic institutions since 2002, there is growing awareness at all levels of Afghan society that economic and social progress requires contribution by all active and able human resources including women.

INSTITUTIONAL FRAMEWORK TO ADVANCE WOMEN'S STATUS

The Ministry of Women's Affairs (MoWA) was established by the Bonn Agreement and was tasked by the interim and transitional governments of Afghanistan with responsibility for advancing the role of women. Although new as a Ministry, a precedent institution for the promotion of women has existed since 1928, when 'Society for the Protection of Women' was established. As a quasi-government body, the 'Society' has faded or flourished with the changing values of the Afghan political leadership throughout the 20th Century.

The MoWA carries responsibility for leading and coordinating government efforts to advance the role of women in all spheres of social life so that gender disparities are reduced and progress towards gender equality is gradually achieved. Ultimately it aims to lead and coordinate inter-ministerial gender policy and strategy development, but recognizes a prior need to build understanding and capacity throughout the government for gender analysis to promote broad-based ownership and commitment. Its key functions are advocacy, technical support, coordination, and monitoring of progress. It attempts to influence sector strategies, lobby national institutions, and support project implementation.

HEALTH

Women in Afghanistan have an extraordinarily high risk of dying during pregnancy and childbirth and the highest maternal mortality rate in the world. Pre-natal care, maternal health care facilities and trained health personnel are virtually non-existent in large parts of the country, contributing to a very high percentage of preventable maternal and child deaths. Besides the lack of access to and quality of health services, other factors such as lack of adequate food, shelter and clean water, low marriage age, high fertility rate and lack of spacing of child births contribute to the extremely poor health of Afghan women.

The root causes of the alarming health indicators in Afghanistan are poverty and the two decades of warfare that stalled economic and social progress and led to destruction of livelihoods and high levels of disability. This situation has had a particularly negative impact on the health and mortality of women and children, but there does not appear to be any evidence of deliberate gender-based discrimination within the health sector - the exception being the Taliban insisting on separate medical facilities for males and females, which increased the de facto differences in service provision to men and women.

However, factors such as the prevailing poverty and lack of health facilities and trained staff, along with the predominant cultural attitudes related to *purdah* norms, have had a devastating effect on women's reproductive health. This chapter focuses on the material circumstances and constraints affecting women's health in terms of access to and availability of health.

MATERNAL AND CHILD MORTALITY

Surveys conducted in 2002 by UNICEF and the U.S. Centers for Disease Control and Prevention in four provinces of Afghanistan estimated a maternal mortality rate (MMR) of 1,600 per 100,000 live births. There are indications of large variations across geographical areas; Kabul for example, had an estimated MMR of 400 per 100,000 while Badakhshan with 6,500 per 100,000 had the highest MMR ever reported globally. In comparison, the MMR is 500 in Pakistan and only 76 in Iran.

The proportion of deaths of women that were due to maternal causes ranged from 16% in Kabul, where at least one maternity hospital was functional at the time of the survey, to 64% in Badakhshan, where health care access was profoundly limited. While the lifetime risk of maternal death is 1 in 15, the UNICEF/CDC study also showed that when the mother of a newborn infant dies, the child has only one chance in four of surviving until its first birthday. Available health data indicate that while the present health situation in Afghanistan is very poor, for the larger part of the population there has not been an actual deterioration as compared to pre-war times.

Despite of the devastating effect of the war and recent drought on all public services in Afghanistan, its pre-war health statistics were even worse. The under-5 mortality has fallen from 360 in 1960 to 260 in 1990 and 257 in 2002. Likewise, maternal mortality rate has fallen from 3,070 per 100 000 in 1978 to the present 1,600, and life expectancy has increased from 38 years (1970) to 43 today. Overall, there have been modest improvements since the 1970s, which presumably are largely due to the scattered service provisions by NGO during the years of conflict.

More than 80% of functional health facilities have some form of NGO involvement, but the coverage is far from even, with a concentration in the urban areas and areas near the Pakistan border. The key point is that in terms of its social indicators, especially female social indicators, Afghanistan has not participated in the dramatic improvements that have occurred over the past several decades in most developing countries, even very poor countries. Thus Afghanistan has fallen much further behind most of the rest of the world and hence is starting from an extremely low base in terms of progressing toward the Millennium Development Goals (MDGs).

A study in Herat province concludes that the extraordinarily high number of deaths of women during pregnancy and childbirth are largely preventable. They are a direct consequence of the very young marriage age for women and girls (according to UNIFEM, 54% of girls under the age of 18 are married), poor health and nutrition, too-frequent childbearing, and virtually no access to gynecological and obstetrical services. Small, anemic mothers with undeveloped pelvic bones are at greater risk of obstructed births with devastating consequences for both mother and baby, and they may not withstand pregnancy or the usual blood loss during delivery. Other studies similarly point out that 40% of child deaths are due to the preventable causes of diarrhea and acute respiratory diseases.

There are no national figures for average marriage age for girls, but in this study it was found to be the age of 15 (range 5-39). The Tufts University study based on *NRVA* data informs us that 16% of girls are married under the age of 15; while 52% are married by the time they become 18 years old. The main causes of maternal mortality are hemorrhage (24%) and obstructed labor (32%). To this should be added the extremely high prevalence of anemia (*MICS2000* recorded 55%-91% for the Southern and Eastern regions). More than 90% of women give birth at home and most of these births occur without the assistance of a trained health attendant.

Even if a primary health care clinic is available, 70% of these are unable to provide even basic mother and child services, while 90% of hospitals do not have the complete equipment to perform C-sections. Furthermore, there is widespread reluctance to let women be treated by male health workers, particularly in the case of obstetrical and gynecological matters. In this context, the fact that in 2002 nearly 40% of basic health facilities did not have female health care workers, only 24% had at least one female physician, 21% had at least one female nurse, and 20% had at least one midwife becomes even more salient.

Where female health workers are present, women's utilization of health care facilities increases dramatically, as is the case in the MSF-supported clinic in Baharak (Badakhshan

Province), staffed with two male and two female doctors. Such clinics in Eshkeshem and Dashta Barchi reported similarly high usage by women. Even with availability of female medical staff, pregnant women may not receive the necessary medical attention. In Eshkeshm it was reported that most problems during birth were taken care of by relatives or by a mullah, who would provide amulets or written verses from the Koran.

In the same vein, the Herat study found that besides women's limited access to health facilities, other factors also contributed to the very high incidence of maternal mortality. These included:

1. Women and their families do not know the warning signs of potentially lethal conditions during pregnancy and childbirth and therefore cannot avert potential complications;
2. Women often cannot afford to pay for health care services even when they know they are in danger; and
3. Lack of transportation makes it impossible for the sick woman to reach the health clinic in time.

Since women normally would consult their male family members about seeking medical care, and in any case may need their assistance for the travel to a health clinic, the lack of male knowledge and understanding of reproductive health care is as important an obstacle as women's own lack of awareness. However, the massive rehabilitation effort undertaken since 2002 is beginning to show results. The first comprehensive study on women and children conducted by the Afghanistan Central Statistics Office and UNICEF in 2003 revealed that estimated infant mortality has fallen from 165 to 115 deaths per 1000 live births and under-5 mortality from 257 to 172 deaths per 1,000 live births.

Furthermore, provision of the Basic Package of Health Services (BPHS) has expanded to about 60% of the population, and 95% of children are vaccinated against measles and polio. Female staffs are now available at 60% of health facilities. While these are very positive indicators, there is still a long way to go.

GENDER DIFFERENCES IN MORTALITY

According to the newly published *National Human Development Report* (2004), life expectancy at birth in Afghanistan is 44.5 years which is about the lowest in the world, comparable to Niger, Burkina Faso and Guinea-Bissau and only Sierra Leone is lower. The neighboring countries of Pakistan and Iran have life expectancy at birth at 60.8 and 70.1 years respectively. Nevertheless, women do have an overall biological advantage in survival at birth, but this survival advantage is extremely small and in the region, only Nepal ranks below Afghanistan, in that respect.

The sex ratio in South Asian countries (with the exception of Sri Lanka), favors men - the starkest indicator of women's poorer health status compared to men's. In Afghanistan too, there are 94 women to every 1000 men - but the sex ratio is the same as in Bangladesh and India. Thus, Afghanistan falls well within the regional patterns in overall gender differences in mortality.

However, survey data from Badghis on age-specific death rates shows that women's death rates in Afghanistan in the reproductive period are particularly sobering and - as women are almost three times as likely as men to die in the 15-49 age group. There is little information on gender discrimination within the household in matters of nutrition and access to health care, but it seems that breastfeeding is discontinued earlier for girls than for boys: breastfeeding was discontinued by age 12-15 months for 6.7% of boys, but for 11% of girls.

FERTILITY AND FAMILY PLANNING

In Afghanistan, there is a marked preference among parents for a newborn to be a boy rather than a girl, which is also a common feature in all the neighboring countries. In the 1970s, before the conflict started, a ratio of almost 2 to 1 favoring boys was reported, and rural women reportedly desired two times as many offspring (boys and girls) as their urban counterparts. In a number of countries of East and South Asia, this has resulted in sex selective abortion resulting in a dramatic shortfall of women.

Fortunately there are no such indications from Afghanistan, where the technology for sex determinations is not yet available, and where the high fertility rate recorded, partly a result of the young marriage age, reflects the fact that numerous children (boys and girls) are seen as a blessing. Having many children functions as a social safety net in a country with no welfare system, related to power in a society where differences are settled through violence and provision of livelihood support by offspring.

Children are important as a female status symbol since a woman's status in the family improves according to the number of children and especially boys she has borne, and failure to conceive is sufficient grounds for a husband to demand divorce. Recent surveys among Pashtun women noted that the desired number of children ranged from seven to ten, while economic considerations and deterioration in the mother's health have been found to be common reasons for men and women to limit their fertility. The current fertility rate is recorded as 6.8, and although high it still constitutes a reduction from the pre-conflict rate of 7.7 recorded in 1960.

To this picture should be added accounts of a virtual 'baby boom' in the refugee camps, where Dupree reported fertility rate of 13.6. It is not known how comprehensive and representative a survey is behind these data, but an increase in fertility rates during a period of war and conflict is however not unusual in any culture. The high fertility rate results in high annual population growth roughly estimated at 3.8% per annum during 1992-2002 according to one source. This is problematic at the individual household level due to the strain it exerts on maternal health and on the economic resources and well-being of the household. The *NRVA* survey reveals that family size is inversely related to per-capita expenditures, and poverty as such also correlates with schooling, literacy and health.

At the national level, rapid population growth will reduce the benefits to the people (in terms of average per-capita income) of any given rate of economic growth. Family planning was introduced to Afghanistan in 1970 when the Department of Family Planning was established in Kabul, with branches extending to 20 provinces a year later. Women in particular did recognize that many child-births and lack of spacing of births took a heavy toll on their health, while the male response to family planning was considerably cooler. The contraceptive prevalence rate reported in 1972/73 by UNFPA was 2%. During the 1980s, little attention was paid to birth control measures, and the Department of Family Planning was closed down with the advent of the *mujahedin* government in 1992.

In this context the very low prevalence of contraception reported recently is not surprising, and it probably reflects both the lack of awareness of and lack of access to contraceptive methods. While contraceptive prevalence in Afghanistan is only 1/5 of the prevalence in Pakistan and 1/11 of the prevalence in Bangladesh, recent surveys have indicated that women in Afghanistan and their husbands are keen to limit family size. Where women do want to limit fertility, access to contraception is the most important determinant.

Estimates of contraceptive prevalence vary substantially, and as in other countries, regional differences are great, with 2% contraceptive prevalence in the South-eastern region compared to 8.4% in the Eastern region are reported by the MICS 2000. While data on reproductive decision-making is lacking in Afghanistan, available evidence seems to show that while women may openly have little say with respect to the number of children they bear, in fact they do have a high unmet need for contraception. The Tufts University survey in 2003 also reported high interest in birth control among women in Badghis, Herat, Kabul, Kandahar and Nangarhar, and several women stated that their husbands would support their use of contraception.

Even more striking is a survey of 360 women in 12 areas of Kabul by Terre des homes, which reported that 98% women expressed interest in receiving contraceptives and 96% confirmed that their husbands would agree with family planning methods. Knowledge of family planning and its use vary considerably between rural and urban areas. According to the MICS 2003, 21% of urban but only for 6% of rural women below 50 years of age reported using contraception. Available figures also indicate that the awareness and usage of contraceptive methods are far higher in the Western part of the country than in other areas.

Thus, women in Herat province are more likely to use contraception than those in Kabul, and even very poor and under-serviced provinces like Farah and Nimroz figure well above the national average when it comes to use of contraceptive methods. Even a very gender conservative province like Kandahar ranks high in terms of both awareness and use of contraception. The reason may be that many Afghans from the western areas were refugees in Iran, where they may have been exposed to the Iranian family planning campaign. (This may also explain why Bamiyan Province in Central Afghanistan ranks high regarding awareness of contraception, since many Shi'as from the central areas chose to become refugees in Iran).

POVERTY, CONFLICT AND GENDER: OTHER EFFECTS ON HEALTH

In the Health Sector, a picture of a largely under-serviced rural population is apparent. In 1976-77, there were a total of 176 government-licensed trained nurse-midwives in the whole of Afghanistan, and of these 150 were in Kabul Province alone. Today the ratio of basic health centers to population ranges from approximately one per 40,000 people in the central and eastern regions to approximately one per 200,000 in the south. Nineteen districts have no health facilities at all.

In 38% of the rural districts countrywide, the majority of people (>50%) have no access to even the most rudimentary forms of healthcare. The slightly more than half of the respondents in the Tufts University survey in Badghis, Herat, Kabul, Kandahar and Nanagarhar provinces, who were able to access some form of health care had to spend on average three hours of travel time to reach the health facility. Hence patients tend to wait until their health problems become severe before they travel to medical centers. The uneven geographical distribution of health facilities is made even worse by the uneven distribution of female health workers.

In 2002 there was one female nurse per 58,988 of population in Balkh Province, while there was one female nurse per 470,500 populations in Ghor Province. In Wardak, 59,000 members of the population shared one midwife, while 475,100 people shared one midwife in Helmand. In Nimroz, Paktika and Khost Provinces, there was not a single basic health facility providing delivery care services with a female physician, doctor's assistant, nurse or midwife.

More than half of all hospitals in Afghanistan are located in Kabul and therefore serve only about one fifth of the entire population. According to WHO, approximately 2,700 of the 3,900 physicians and 600 of the 990 midwives work in Kabul, leaving the remainder of the country with few trained health care professionals. In fact, it was recently estimated that a trained health care provider attended fewer than 8% of deliveries countrywide, and there is one doctor per 1,000 populations in Kabul, whereas there is only one per 100,000 populations in Bamiyan. In the case of rural health facilities which are fortunate enough to have a medical officer, he/she may only have limited medical education completed decades ago.

The number of doctors plus the 7,000 medical students may exceed the number of trained community health workers in the country, which means that the primary health pyramid has been stood on its head, with a focus on curative care, whereas notions of public health are poorly developed. The congruence of poverty, conflict and prevailing gender norms has also had other adverse effects on the health of women and men. The extreme anti-women policies of the Taliban regime from the mid-1990s to 2001 and the years of conflict have, for example, increased women's risk of mental diseases.

For example, study of maternal mortality in Herat points out that a large percentage of Afghan women suffer from major depression or other mental health problems related to trauma and/or the suffering of losses in their lives. Evidence from Medica Mondiale, a German-based international organisation supporting women in war and crisis situations, reports that a Herat hospital last year recorded 160 cases of attempted suicide among girls and women between the ages of 12 and 50. This is widely recognized by aid workers as being an underestimation of the problem due to reporting bias in favor of urban areas.

Nutritional deprivation stemming from food insecurity and issues of occupational health are some of the other issues of concern. The MICS 2000 reported 14% of children as being severely underweight and 25% as severely stunted, although gender disaggregated data is not available. In 2002 UNICEF and CDC conducted a child nutritional assessment in Badghis, covering 507 households, where chronic malnutrition was reported for 62% of boys and 54% of girls, while prevalence of acute malnutrition was 6-7% for both.

Finally, specific workrelated problems affect women and men differently. For instance, girls who work at carpet looms from an early age face problems of neurological and eye related problems due to the constant high concentration required. Other evidence on the health effects of conflict and poverty is lacking, and this is a critical area for further research.

INNOVATIVE PROGRAMMES CARRIED OUT BY NGOS

NGOs have shown the way to effective health service delivery in the difficult conditions of Afghanistan, albeit on a small scale. A variety of approaches have been adopted to provide access for rural women to reproductive health information and services. Mobile clinics are used by agencies like Relief International (RI), which serves five districts of Nangarhar province traveling from its capital in Jalalabad. The Afghanistan Institute of Learning (AIL) covers three districts of Kabul province from its Mir Bacha Kot based unit.

Both agencies integrate direct care with preventive approaches implemented by non-health professionals in order to optimize outcomes for women. Over the past five years AIL has trained 10,000 female teachers to provide health education to women in their communities. Capitalizing on its relationship with the Ministry of Education (as an education provider) its mobile clinics also implement specialized health seminars in schools for both adults and for children. Relief International expands its outreach for preventive health education through literacy teachers as well as community health workers, and focuses its mobile clinic in those districts where women are participating in a non-formal education programme.

POLICY IMPLICATIONS

Afghanistan's health indicators are among the worst in the world, in particular, when it comes to child health and women's reproductive health. Under-five mortality rate of 257, infant mortality rate of 165, and estimated maternal mortality rate of 16 (all per 1000 live births); rate of chronic malnutrition (moderate or severe stunting) around 50%; and very high rates of disability due to polio, cerebral palsy, and conflict (including landmines) are figures that tell the sorry state of affairs. Recent surveys have revealed that almost half of all deaths among women of reproductive age are a result of pregnancy and childbirth - and that more than ¾ of these deaths are preventable.

Among children, diarrhea, acute respiratory infections and vaccine preventable illnesses likely account for 60% of deaths, and among adults tuberculosis results in an estimated 15,000 deaths per year, with 70% of detected cases being among women. Life expectancy is estimated at 43 years. A range of factors contributes to this situation.

On the supply side it is:

- Lack of access to basic health facilities - only 40% of the population is in the coverage areas of basic health facilities, and only 9% of rural households surveyed in 2003 reported a health facility in their village
- Lack of female staff at the existing facilities particularly in rural areas

- Strong rural-urban disparity in availability of health facilities
- Lack of roads, transport and security reduce mobility and access
- Public health system, including provision of community health workers, is highly underdeveloped compared to the curative care in the primary health system
- Lack of clean drinking water and sanitation facilities
- Lack of access to family planning information and contraceptive methods

Social factors, which negatively affect women's health and their inability to access proper healthcare, are:

- Low marriage age resulting in too many and too frequent child births
- Poverty Reluctance to let women seek medical assistance from male health workers
- Lack of awareness of maternal health care among men and women
- Insufficient awareness of health hygiene and nutrition
- Lack of awareness of family planning

WORK AND EMPLOYMENT

The economy of Afghanistan has always been agriculture-based, and it is estimated that up to 80% of the population live in the rural areas. Contributing an estimated 53% to GDP and 67% to the labor force in 2003, agriculture (including crops, livestock, forestry and fishery) is central to the Afghan economy. Agricultural and related activities are a major vehicle for women's participation in the economy. Production is dominated mainly by subsistence-oriented family holdings, with a well-defined division of labor based on age and gender. Locations, cropping patterns, ethnic affiliation and economic and educational background also have implications for the specific division of labor within a given household, since communities differ regarding women's participation in agriculture.

Horticulture generally involves women more than grain production, and poor households require greater involvement of women in income earning activities than do more wealthy households. This chapter discusses women's contribution to agriculture and livestock production and regional variation, as well as women's other income generating activities, along with the various social factors affecting them. It is demonstrated that women play an important role in all dimensions of agricultural production - in certain regions women's time input equals men's, while in other regions traditions restrict their work to the household where they are involved in crop processing and are in charge of household maintenance and reproductive activities.

In most cases women's labor is non-monetized, but they make large labor contributions to a range of marketed products such as dried fruits, opium, fuel wood, dairy products and handicrafts. Women's involvement in the formal sector has grown since the 1960s, mainly as civil servants in the health and education sectors. Currently, close to one-third of all teachers are female, but many more are required to ensure increased enrollment of girls. In the health sector, an estimated 40% of health facilities lack female staff, which along with the shortage of rural health facilities constitutes a major constraint to delivering much needed health services to the female half of the population.

Unlike in the case of education and health, the gender and employment picture in Afghanistan is similar to that in other parts of the South Asia region - particularly Pakistan and northern India. Women's labor force participation rates in Afghanistan are comparable to the rest of the region at 35.8 % - lower than in Bangladesh (42.5%), Nepal (40.5%) and Sri Lanka (36.9%), but higher than in India (32.5%) and Pakistan (29.5%).

While gender disaggregated data are not available by sector of employment, the likelihood is that this relatively high level of female labor force participation is due to the needs of an agrarian and pastoral economy. Second, poverty drives women's employment in Afghanistan, as it does in other South Asian countries, and high poverty rates are no doubt responsible for high female labor force participation.

Agriculture and Women's Work

In rural Afghanistan, as elsewhere in the region, there are distinct male and female roles in the rural economy. Evidence from surveys in Laghman, Ghazni, Badakhshan, Bamiyan, Paktia, Helmand, Faryab and Saripul confirms that women and girls engage in a number of farm based activities ranging from seed bed preparation, weeding, horticulture, and fruit cultivation to a series of post-harvest crop processing activities such as cleaning and drying vegetables, fruits and nuts for domestic use and for marketing.

In a survey in Badakhshan, it was observed that women carry out 37% of the household work, while men do only 15%. Girls carry out 27% of domestic activities and boys do only 21%. Turning to the agricultural activities, women and men's contribution in terms of time allocation was found to be almost equal - but whereas women were found to be dominant within the domestic tasks, men were dominant as regards agriculture and livestock. There were considerable variations among the various districts, but in general women tend to play a greater role in agricultural and livestock production in Badakhshan than is the case in the southern and eastern parts of Afghanistan.

Badakhshan is also known for comparatively more equitable gender relations than most other areas. The study of Badakhshan also point towards the different nature of men's and women's agricultural activities, which presumably would apply to other regions as well. Male activities such as land preparation, planting/sowing, and fertilizer application are one-time jobs and usually accomplished within a specific, limited time. In comparison, female activities such as weeding are recurrent daily activities, lasting from the time that the seed is planted until it is harvested. In spite of spending the same amount of time on agricultural activities, women's work in general tends to be less visible and of lower value compared to men's.

Often women's products are bartered rather than sold, and this is both a cause and a consequence of their perceived lower contribution to the rural economy. This attitude even extends to a number of products produced by women, which can only be exchanged in kind but not sold, since selling them would be considered shameful. Non-monetary exchange relations between households also contribute to social networking and cohesion, and are thus an important aspect of building social capital. A comparative study of three villages in Laghman illustrates women's work in another regional context, and although the overall picture is similar there are local variations in the degree of women's participation.

A combination of factors was found to affect women's participation in agricultural production, not only in these specific communities. Women in poor households, or households with a low worker/dependent ratio, tend to participate in more agricultural tasks outside the home. If the need is great enough, women may, in spite of the prevalent social norms, even engage in wage work on other peoples' land. This is not a new phenomenon but has been an option for poor households for many years. Many smaller surveys and case studies have indicated that women contribute in a significant manner to the family income - but that variations between regions and income groups are so large that simple generalizations should be avoided. The *NRVA* survey now provides a far broader quantitative basis for analysis.

According to Maletta (2003), 55.5% of the wealth groups98 reported women having worked during the past year in some gainful activity (excluding housekeeping, and other 'non-economic' activities, including food for work or other relief activity), with the highest frequency in the North, Northeast and West. A closer look at the figures reveals that averages are not very informative in view of the huge variations - from about 80% or more of women in the North, Northeast and West down to less than 14% in the South.

IMPLICATIONS FOR WOMEN'S WORK

The role of women in agricultural production is largely determined by the life cycle of the household, the location of household fields and other reproductive and productive tasks that women undertake during the agricultural year. The availability of sufficient labor within the household can often mean that women are not required to participate in cultivation outside the family compound. However, widows, women with young children, or married daughters will often be required to assist with the cultivation of particular labor-intensive crops.

These observations are largely confirmed in the study Gender Roles in Agriculture in five villages in Faryab and Saripul, where Grace furthermore sums up, "It appears that the richer the household, the less the women work on land. Also, there appears to be a stigma attached to women working on land, as it denotes that the family is poor." This observation can safely be assumed to have general validity all over Afghanistan. With the *NRVA*, there are now large-scale comprehensive data available, which confirm the general picture emerging from the case studies of various regions.

Across all regions and social groups, it is a cherished ideal that the men of the household should be the breadwinners, while women take care of domestic chores. However, most households cannot live up to this ideal, and women contribute in a variety of ways to the family's upkeep. But the ideal is reflected in the relative frequency of female gainful work among different wealth groups, with poor and very poor groups of women showing higher frequencies, 60% as compared to 46% among the better-off groups. The percentages are much higher in the North, Northeast and West than in other regions. Some specific occupations like domestic service are highly concentrated in the "very poor" group. Other activities, however, are more or less equally present in all the wealth groups.

There is an inverse relationship between wealth and work, i.e. the frequency of work increases as wealth decreases. But some activities have a reverse pattern - they are practiced more frequently by those with a medium or higher level of wealth, such as embroidery and tailoring of clothes. There is thus a kind of stratification of various activities between the upper wealth group and the very poor. Embroidery is practiced three times more frequently among the richer than among the very poor, while domestic service is at the other extreme: for every 100 very poor groups reporting it, it is reported by only six better-off groups, i.e. 1 in 16.

The definition of 'economic activity' excludes the exchange of labor and products between households, which women in particular are engaged in. It also seems to exclude the post-harvest processing of crops (drying/cleaning/preserving), which is a predominately female domain - and it excludes the vital role women in the South play regarding a household's contracting of poppy harvesters, for whom three solid daily meals are part of their wage packet. Different regional practices regarding female 'economic' activities particularly the South representing a tradition where women's activities mainly take place within the four walls of the household. While the relative proportions between regions are probably realistic, the absolute figures thus underestimate women's 'gainful activities'.

Fruit Cultivation

The cropping pattern in a given locality has a considerable impact on women's participation in agricultural production, with grain production having the least female involvement and horticulture (vegetables, melons etc.), fruits and nuts in general including large labor input from girls and women. These are major cash crops, which counted for around half of all export earnings in the 1970s, when Afghanistan was the world's largest exporter of dried fruit.

Opium

Currently opium is the biggest cash crop in Afghanistan, and women play an important role in the cultivation of opium poppy in both the northern and eastern regions of Afghanistan. They are involved at various stages of opium poppy cultivation including planting and weeding, thinning, lancing the capsules, collecting the opium, clearing the fields, breaking the capsules and removing the seeds, cleaning the seeds, and processing byproducts such as oil and soap. Women's role in cultivation is more visible and more valued in opium production than for example in wheat production - and both women and children get paid for their work in collection of opium resin in Badakhshan.

However, in the southern region which tends to be more conservative and where land ownership is more concentrated, women's participation in opium poppy cultivation is restricted to the task of preparing food and drink for itinerant opium poppy harvesters. But in both the east and the south, poppy harvest is a labor- intensive time for women as well as men. Given the size of the hired workforce, the preparation of this food and drink is reported to increase women's workload significantly.

The low opportunity cost associated with women's labor tends to make labor-intensive crops, such as opium poppy, a more attractive option for the household and poppy cultivation also involves widespread use of reciprocal labor. While it is often assumed that the burden of many women find their workloads increased, by working on their own land, the land of their relatives, and preparing food for the *ashar* labor. Indeed, in the eastern region, women expressed a preference for the use of hired labor over that of *ashar* due to the fact that hired labor did not require food. The public role of women in reciprocal labor arrangements for opium poppy cultivation highlights the importance of unpaid labor in the production of poppy.

Supplementary Incomes

The livelihood of most rural households consists of a mosaic of jobs, such as crop production, livestock, cutting of wood, labor and a number of other small-scale activities, and women frequently contribute with economic activities beyond agriculture. In mountainous villages, for example in Laghman, cutting and selling wood is an important seasonal activity for men and women alike, providing income for the household during the winter. Similarly, pistachio trees growing on government land on the Northern plains were considered a public good which contributed much needed cash to rural households through the joint efforts of all household members.

The district government administration controlled access to this good and at harvest time announced publicly when the various villages of the district were allowed to go and collect pistachios in a specified locality. All men and young boys would go for days to collect the pistachios, and on their return to the village, all of the women and children would work for days and nights de-shelling the pistachios, after which men would sell them to middlemen in the nearby bazaar. As a result of the conflict and the drought the pistachio forests are said to be depleted.

Livestock

Most rural households also keep livestock, mainly for domestic consumption of meat, milk, wool, eggs, etc., and occasionally for sale. The pastoral economy contributes significantly to the national economy. Women and children are the main tenders of animals. Boys are usually in charge of taking the animals for grazing while women and girls collect fodder. Hence, while women have a significant responsibility for animals, their livestock management in most areas is centered on the home, taking care of newborn and sick animals, milking, collecting fodder and stable feeding. In some of the northeastern mountainous areas in Panjshir and Badakhshan, the women play a far wider role in livestock management and may go to summer pastures without their families to tend animals and produce dairy products, even on contract for neighbors.

Most rural households have some animals. The main production of livestock prior to the conflict and drought was by the pastoral nomads, with a gender and age division of labor broadly similar to the settled rural communities. Before the drought the pastoral economy contributed significantly to the national economy, with carpets/rugs, skins and wool being major export products. The carpets and rugs are primarily produced by women, who also play a major role in the preparation of the wool, as well as participating in the processing of the hides and skins and sheep casings.

SOCIAL AND OCCUPATIONAL STRATIFICATION

The socioeconomic status of the household determines the types of work that women do. At one end of the spectrum, the poorest women engage in manual agricultural labor or wage work outside the home (if available), while at the other end women from better-off families engage in sedentary, home-based activity. Overall, a recent survey reports that over 55% of women work in at least one economic activity, and the difference by wealth group for women engaging in any activity is relatively small (46% for the richest and 61% for the poorest women). Thus there is an inverse relationship between wealth and work, i.e. the frequency of the work increases as wealth decreases.

But some activities have a reverse pattern - they are practiced more frequently by those with a medium or higher level of wealth, there is thus stratification among various activities, and the richest are three times more likely to practice embroidery than the poorest, while the poorest are 16 times more likely than the richest to work in domestic service.

Weaving and handicrafts are almost equally practiced across the socioeconomic divide and are among the 'desirable' activities for women (since a girl in any case is expected to do needlework for her trousseau), and which are socially acceptable to monetize, i.e. to produce for sale. Farm work, gathering wood and especially domestic service are practiced overwhelmingly by the very poor out of necessity - the first two because they go beyond women's accepted domestic chores and entail involvement in the male-dominated public sphere, and the third because it involves relations of servitude and inferiority and thus is socially degrading.

GENDER WAGE GAPS

Almost no economy pays equal wages to men and women, even for the same work, and Afghanistan is no exception. In agriculture, women receive a fraction of the wages that men do, ranging from 50% to 60% for specific tasks. The *NRVA* provides very useful information in this regard. These wage gaps are indicative of the value placed on women's work and on the social context of female poverty, e.g. in case of female headed households. The *NRVA* survey results show that the wage ratios (women/men) are 51% for planting, 61% for harvesting, and 50% for other farm work. In the case of non-farm occupations, the wage paid to women for making handicrafts is 41% of the male salary, and for weaving the ratio is 53% - men being paid US$1.17 per day for weaving while women receive only $0.62 per day.

A woman gathering wood fetches 53% of the male pay - US$0.81 per day as compared to her male counterpart who is paid US$1.54 per day. In the case of domestic work, women are even paid less than children - an average of US$0.59 per day, while a child doing the same work earns US$0.74. There is no obvious explanation for this gap - but may perhaps relate to fact that children are subject to fewer social restrictions on their mobility than women. A woman employed in domestic work for others earns 28% of a male construction worker's and 41% of a male shepherd's wage.

PROPERTY RIGHTS AND CONTROL OVER RESOURCES

High labor force participation rates do not automatically grant women control over resources nor access to property rights, as seen in many mountainous villages, for example in Laghman Women's economic activities in the village can be divided into those which contribute to the household economy but where the income is controlled by the men (activities where women contribute basically their labor), and those activities which generate income and the income is controlled by the women themselves. The use of income, if any, from agricultural produce is in most families controlled by men. Afghanaid's studies from Badakhshan mention that in spite of men and women's equal time spent on agriculture and livestock, the control of expenditures is the men's prerogative.

The same applies to the income generated through the sale of wood which was the second most important source of income recorded from studies in mountain villages in Laghman. Likewise, livestock was also being owned either by the household (i.e. owned jointly between men and women) or by men. Only chickens were specifically reported as being owned exclusively and de facto by women. Local custom regarding women's inheritance rights differ between ethnic groups and regions.

In a study of land relations in Faryab province, Wily notes that while cases of female inheritance were recorded particularly among Tajiks, no instances of widows inheriting land or houses were found among the Arab and Pashtun communities. Female land ownership is not common among Uzbeks, either. On the other hand, in Laghman female landowners are quite common, as reported from the study of three villages in Alingar. About 50% of reported landowners were female, apparently acquiring land through inheritance.

In reality, the women seemed to have little control over the land: The de jure position is that women do own land, while the de facto position is that they rarely exercise their right to land as they stand to lose too much if they do so, a situation which seems largely similar to communities in North Afghanistan.

Wily noted from Bamiyan that "(W) women's land ownership is not a live issue". In a survey of 15 villages only ten cases (2.5%) of women owning land were recorded. While not all of the female landowners were widows, a common trend seemed to be that sisters surrendered the land inherited from their father to a brother.

One woman explained the rationale as follows: "Girls must get land to meet the requirements of Islam, but they are not expected to keep it. If they keep it, they cannot expect their brothers to care for them if they face problems. My brother took my sister presents. He bought her a sheep and clothes. He praised her. At the same time he called us and the elders to witness in writing that she had passed the land over to him."

URBAN EMPLOYMENT

In urban areas women's employment outside the domestic sphere has always been limited and subject to severe restrictions. In 1975-76 approximately 5.6% of government employees were female, while in the industrial sector only 1,536 out of a total 36,875 employees were women. The fertilizer and electricity establishment in Mazar-i Sharif employed the largest number of women; in addition factories which processed foods and beverages or produced cotton cloth also had considerable numbers of female workers. During the PDPA government, the female labor force in the cities increased and women were employed in all major government departments, in addition to the police force, the army, business and industry.

Women taught, studied and acted as judges in the Family Court, dealing with issues relating to divorce, custody of children and other family matters. When the Taliban assumed power and initially prohibited all female employment, it was estimated that in Kabul city there were some 40,000 women in public service. They accounted for 70% of all the teachers in Kabul, about 50% of civil servants and an estimated 40% of medical doctors. Professions such as medical doctors, teachers and any office bound work such as administration or engineering design were generally considered 'appropriate' for women in the urban context and could be seen as an extension of women's roles as mothers and care givers in the home.

But the Taliban initiated wholesale dismissal of female government employees - resulting in international protest in 1996; a compromise was reached whereby women could draw their salaries without working. However, in 1999 the Report of the UN Secretary General on the situation of women and girls in Afghanistan noted reports of the widespread dismissal of female civil servants in a move to cut government spending. The Special Advisor on Gender Issues and Advancement noted that by mid-2000, there were a total of 5,874 Afghan women employed by the international assistance community in Afghanistan (including 1,020 doctors and health workers, 2,066 traditional birth attendants, and 900 WFP bakery staff in Mazar-i Sharif and Jalalabad). There are only limited data available on the post-Taliban representation of women in the civil service.

According to 2003 data from the Central Statistics Office, 21% of all permanent government employees were women. The available evidence on educational qualifications suggests that these women are significantly less educated than male civil servants. Current labor market opportunities for women are very limited in urban areas, and this contributes significantly to urban poverty. Typical employment for unskilled women is domestic work. In the female-headed households surveyed, 52% of women had been working infrequently in Kabul and elsewhere, sewing, embroidering or washing clothes for others. In the 48% of female-headed households where women were not working themselves, their young sons (under 15) were working sporadically as daily wage labor for minimal returns.

In 27% of the male-headed households, women were working as well as men. Women's access to the urban labor market is constrained by historical circumstances, low skills, limited opportunities, stringent cultural norms, occupational sex segregation and a number of demographic factors of which availability of childcare is an important part. According to an IRC survey, up to 40% of interviewed women referred to lack of child care as a constraint to their participation in the labor market. Kinder gardens were first introduced in 1980 as part of the Soviet-inspired Early Childhood Development Programme, where facilities attached to schools, government offices or factories provided nursery care, preschool, and kinder garden for children (3 months to 7 years).

By 1990 there were more than 270 preschools and 2,300 teachers caring for over 21,000 children, mainly in Kabul. Like other institutions, the Kinder gardens closed down during the turmoil of the 1990s following the withdrawal of women from the labor market. In response to complaints from women in government service, Kinder gardens have been reintroduced in a number of ministries. In response to complaints from women in government service, Kindergartens have been reintroduced in a number of ministries during the past several years. In addition to some opportunities in wage employment, women in the urban economy tend to be employed in the informal sector.

A recent market survey of micro-entrepreneurs in Mazar-i Sharif, Pul-i Khumri, Bamiyan, Herat and Kandahar showed that women are more present in services (beauty parlor, tailoring etc.) and production (carpet weaving mainly) than men. Few women work as middlemen or traders, since that would require that they be in contract with strangers. On average, the women entrepreneurs surveyed employ 4.8 employees while male entrepreneurs employ 2.3 persons, since female dominated activities such as tailoring and carpet weaving tend to be more labor-intensive.

Most employees are family members. Women's activities are small-scale compared to men's, with an investment and working capital 15%-20% of that of men and monthly turnover around 25% of men's. Instability and insecurity were rated by both men and women as obstacles to growth, but women mentioned lack of skills and lack of demand more frequently than men did, as well as 'no good suppliers'. Among both men and women lack of funds was the highest rated obstacle. A study of businesswomen in Kabul concluded that while women are active in the urban economy, among the women surveyed there was relatively low vocational capacity in areas outside of handicrafts and other 'traditional' sectors.

This was underlined by the fact that interviewees with no education constituted the majority of participants at 54%, while 11% had attended primary school, 6% secondary school,

16% high school, and 13% had an advanced education. These Kabul businesswomen thus have a comparatively better educational background than the average woman. The constraints raised by these business women were (a) access to market, (b) difficulty in meeting shopkeepers and making arrangements to buy and sell, and (c) reliance on male relatives to manage the non-production aspects of their businesses.

Location of work for the female entrepreneurs who participated in a credit survey was overwhelmingly (99%) in the home, and as an extension of this, women tended not to view their enterprises as formal businesses. Nearly half of the women entrepreneurs indicated that they control their income, and 40% of women would be able to take a loan without permission from a male relative.

Interestingly, in the focus groups the women who were most actively engaged in the public portions of their businesses (input acquisition, market assessment, negotiation with retailers) were those with well-educated husbands (12th class or higher). Women who cited their largest business constraints as their families' prohibition against their going to the market and engaging in the public portions of business also reported that their male relatives were uneducated, or had only one or two years of education.

FEMALE HEADED HOUSEHOLDS AND VULNERABILITY

In the 1970s, before the conflict, in spite of the high rate of widowhood for women (13.2% as compared to 4.5% for men), female headed households were very rare - 1.1% in urban and 1.2% in rural areas. By contrast, in 1996 it was estimated that there were some 45,000 war widows in Kabul, each supporting an average of six dependants. Current estimates of the prevalence of female headed households (FHH) in Afghanistan range from around 16% in Kabul (Caritas) to between 4% and 20% in three districts in Badakhshan (Afghanaid).

The current high frequency of female-headed households reflects how the prevailing poverty and years of conflict have undermined social networks and traditional mechanisms of mutual social support.

The *NRVA* documents that female-headed households are poorer than average. The proportion of female-headed households in the two poorest quintiles (9.3%) is more than double the level in the highest quintile (3.9%). Per capita expenditures in households headed by a female are 14 percentage points lower than those in households headed by a male. The *NRVA* data also reveal that a higher than average proportion of landless are female headed (15%, nearly double the ratio for the sample as a whole), which may reflect the loss of formal asset entitlements by women to male relatives after the loss of a husband.

This phenomenon highlights a key aspect of the gender dimension of Afghanistan's development challenge and most probably reflects that female-headed households in many cases have lost or do not have a very important human asset (working-age male) and the restrictions against women working outside the household in many rural areas, as well as women's lower human capital (particularly education). In view of the destitution experienced by most widows, the need to expand women's income-generating opportunities is urgent.

POLICY IMPLICATIONS

The striking feature of Afghanistan's economic structure is the dominance of the informal sector. Although it is inherently difficult to estimate the size of the informal economy, it is clear that some 80-90% of economic activity in Afghanistan occurs in the informal sector, which has been largely responsible for the recent economic recovery and dynamism. Exchange services between households are widespread, and women perform a major part of this non-monetized work. However, the traditional role of women in Afghanistan is a constraint to their more equitable participation in economic activities, which is especially hard on the large number of female headed households, for whom eking out an existence without a male breadwinner is very difficult.

In particular, female wage labor is still viewed as a solution of last resort for households in desperate straits, and their wage rates are normally only half the level of men's or less. Women have few marketable skills and generally poor education, with an estimated female literacy rate of 21%. But other constraints should not be underestimated. With high fertility and infant and maternal mortality rates, reproduction and related health issues occupy much of women's time. The absence of many services and the need to produce agricultural products for subsistence also imposes an opportunity cost for women who want to join the labor market. Women often lack ownership, control, and access to productive assets such as land, equipment, and materials, and their legal right to inheritance is usually bypassed.

The lack of working capital (and shortage of credit) reduces opportunities to start activities that require an initial investment. Agriculture and related activities will also in the future be a major vehicle for women's participation in the economy. As part of a demand-driven and community-based approach, women should be explicitly targeted which will reap major benefits in terms of agricultural production and incomes. Within the informal sector women's participation and income-earning possibilities should be increased, while increased female employment in the public sector should be ensured: strengthen women's involvement in agricultural and livestock production in the form of extension and training, credit facilities and expanding marketing opportunities.

Applied research and focused policies that target women as producers in agricultural and livestock production development of socially acceptable skilled and unskilled employment opportunities for women in the urban sector in response to the high level of poor female-headed households formation of cooperation among groups of women involved in informal activities and support in the form of guidance on market acceptability, product handling techniques, marketing methods, and calculation of marketing costs secure women's inheritance and property rights, to promote their potential as producers and to address important aspects of rural vulnerability accelerate implementation of micro-credit schemes (MISFA), with particular focus on women.

Integrate skills enhancement training and vocational training with provision of micro-credit, supported by market surveys and training in account keeping improve targeting of poverty-alleviation programmes to provide minimal safety net to the most vulnerable groups such as female-headed households technological skills upgrading in the traditional handicrafts sectors to increase its income earning and export potential support to businesswomen through access to credit, raw materials, training and markets substantial strengthening of women's employment in the health and education sectors, which will have direct positive effects on girls' school enrollment, women's access to health services, maternal mortality and general child and family health collection of adequate sex-disaggregated data across all sectors to document women's and men's involvement and to enable monitoring of future developments and effects of investments.

5

Work and Identity

Among the alleyways of Dolly, in Indonesia's second-largest city, it is not difficult to find thousands of young women lured by the prospects of a better life working as commercial sex workers (CSWs). "I never chose to be a prostitute. It just happened," Isah, 19, told IRIN, describing her tenure in one of Southeast Asia's largest commercial sex venues. Married and divorced by 17, Isah was easy prey for traffickers, who promised her a well-paid job in the city. "After my divorce, there was no way I could return to my family. I had to escape," she said, only to find herself servicing up to eight men a night for about US$30 per day.

Such stories are common in East Java, Indonesia's most populous province, particularly in rural areas, with thousands of women being trafficked both internally and abroad for prostitution.

In Dolly alone, more than 2,500 women now work as CSWs; a large number of them trafficked. While no official statistics are available, data suggest that 80,000-100,000 women and children are victims of sexual exploitation or have been trafficked for such purposes each year, many to Malaysia and the Middle East, while others are sent to the capital Jakarta or Kalimantan (Borneo), an island rich in timber, coffee and rubber plantations where large numbers of men live alone. An estimated 30 percent of all female sex workers are younger than 18, some as young as 10.

ESCAPE ROUTES

Although some trafficking victims - both inside and outside Indonesia - manage to escape, their numbers remain few. In Malaysia alone, some 900 women seek assistance annually; a figure widely believed to be just 10 percent of the total. "These figures are really just the tip of the iceberg," Jasmina Byrne, the UN Children's Fund (UNICEF) chief of child protection programmes in Jakarta, said. Trafficking is the result of many interrelated factors, say specialists, including a lack of protection mechanisms, which allows unscrupulous agents to work more freely.

Job opportunities are slim in the world's largest archipelago, and migration offers hope for a better future - particularly in rural areas where a large number of people live on or below the poverty line. According to the World Bank, close to 20 percent of the population - the fourth-largest in the world - live below the national poverty line. "Poverty is the driving factor," Diyan Wahyuningsih, coordinator of Genta, a local NGO, in Surabaya, which also runs one of two shelters in the city for trafficking victims, said.

Conditions are particularly bad for young people, but even more so for girls, with fewer opportunities for education and job opportunities. Many see the bright lights of the cities as an escape, but without the necessary knowledge and skills to survive many are exploited.

LEGISLATION

Although the government enacted legislation against human trafficking in 2007, full implementation will take time. Poor law enforcement and corruption lead to few cases being adequately investigated, with offenders regularly going unpunished. "Levels of abuse cases, including prostitution, due to trafficking are increasing," said Waloejo Noegroho, head of the Pusat Pelayanan Terpadu in Surabaya, a government referral office set up to assist children and women survivors of violence, abuse and trafficking, one of 28 such centres in East Java.

"Many of these people are poor and uneducated. They are unaware of their rights and easily tricked," said Yanti Indarsyah, a counsellor at the centre. "Many victims are badly affected and may need long-term therapy".

ADDITIONAL CHALLENGES

According to UNICEF, 60 percent of Indonesian children under-five do not have birth certificates. "If that first protection right - your birth certificate - is not in place, it is very easy to manipulate somebody's identity. You can then present someone as being older than they really are," Byrne said. "This is why you have young girls being trafficked. These girls should not even be allowed to migrate abroad because of their age," she said. UNICEF believes protecting human rights depends on the ability to make the identification and age of a person foolproof, thus reducing the risk of traffickers taking advantage.

Other issues include the continued practice of debt bondage in some places, as well as early marriage and early divorce - all having a contributory effect, as in the case of Isah. The average girl child in the South Asian region symbolizes a combination of suffering, service, and sacrifice from the day she is born to the day she completes her life cycle as a daughter, wife, and mother (Ministry of Women Affairs).

In the South Asian Association for Regional Cooperation (MC) countries (India, Bangladesh, Pakistan, Sri Lanka, Maldives, Bhutan, Nepal), despite the geographical, political, and socio-cultural differences between the countries, the situation of the girl child may be summarized as:.born (if at all) into inequity, die in larger numbers, gets lesser care and protection, receives less education, gets lower pay and inferior treatment at the work place, and has far more chances of becoming sick, pregnant, deserted, abandoned or dead. (WC) With this in mind, a series of consultations were held in South Asia at the regional and national levels focusing particularly on issues related to the girl child.

The purpose was to identify areas for intervention areas in order to develop national action plans. Furthermore, MC officially declared 1990 as the "Year Of the Girl Children and the 1990s as the 'Decade of the Girl Child." Adolescent girlhood has been included in the definition of the "girl children and the age group have been fixed at 0-20 years. Interestingly, empirical evidence suggest that some of the constraints by the girl child in Bhutan, the Maldives, and Sri Lanka relate more to adolescence and unequal opportunities for social mobility and work participation, while those constraints confronting the girl child in India, Bangladesh, Nepal, and Pakistan start before birth and continue into adulthood (UNICEF 1991). Hence, while gender discrimination may be systemic and overt in the latter countries, it may be more subtle in the former. However, the overall situation of deprivation, whether overt or subtle, remains more or less the same throughout the South Asian region.

DEMOGRAPHY AND HEALTH

An extremely important demographic indicator of gender discrimination is the persistence of an adverse sex-ratio in most parts of the South Asian region, particularly in India, Bangladesh, Nepal, and Pakistan. According to Amartya Sen, a noted economist, 77 million women are missing in China and India alone (quoted in Bhasin). The economic situation and food availability are not responsible for it. Countries like India and Pakistan are economically better off than Bhutan in terms of higher Gross National Product but have sex-ratios which declined from 934 females per 1000 males in 1981 to 929 females per 1000 males in 1991 in India (Census of India). Within India itself the lowest sex-ratios were found in Punjab (879: 1000) and Haryana (870: 1 OOO), which are otherwise assumed to be prosperous states (Health Statistics of India). In Jaisalmer (Rajasthan) the sex-ratio is one of the lowest in the world at approximately 550: 1000.

Researchers have attributed such appalling sex-ratios to the practice of female foeticide, female infanticide (Bajpai), health-care and nutritional biases, and mortality and morbidity differentials between genders. In most parts of the South Asian region, the birth of a girl is seldom welcome. More often than not, the girl child receives less food, less nutrition and medical care, and even less love and affection. Such discriminatory practices starting as early as infancy have been well-documented by several studies conducted in Bangladesh, Pakistan, Nepal, and India. These studies show again and again that more male children are immunized and treated in hospitals; mortality due to diarrhoea, respiratory infections, and medes is higher among female children; girls are weaned earlier due to the anxiety to conceive and give birth to a son soon; boys are breast-fed longer; girls eat last after the male members of the family have taken their food; they get less food of poorer quality; nutritious vegetables, fits, eggs, milk, and meat are missing from their diets; and girls are usually brought to hospitals in worse condition than boys.

It is noteworthy that this trend is found in both urban and rural areas as well as across socio-economic groupings (*Sattar*). Thus, during the pre-school years, which are considered by psychologists as the most constructive and developmental phase of an individual's life, the girl child is the most neglected member of the family. This results in the girl child's inadequate mental and physical growth. Anthropogenic measurements (Ministry of Human Resources Development) reveal that girls often have a small pelvis and remain short of statured in adolescence. In most cases, girl children also suffer from serious ailments. Early marriages further aggravate the problem. Clinical malnutrition, cervical cancer, anaemia, and related problems are all connected with early marriage (consummation before 18 years) and early pregnancy before the body is fully mature for procreation. The preference for sons has a powerful influence over the number of pregnancies and hence children, women have to bear.

It has been estimated that preference for a male child adds an average of two or three children per family (Seth and Sen) even at the risk of the life of the mother. Repeated and too frequent pregnancies, particularly among teenage mothers, coupled with lack of access to information and facilities for safe delivery are responsible for babies with low birth weights who are then vulnerable to disease and premature death. In recent years, amniocentesis (though banned) has become common not only in the metropolitan cities of India but also among the rich in rural areas of many northern states. According to one study conducted at the University of Delhi 13,505 pregnant women underwent sex-determination tests in seven clinics in New Delhi in one year alone.

It was observed that most of the female zygotes were aborted after the "without undue anxiety". There is scattered evidence that attests to the prevalence of female infanticide in some parts of India. For instance, amongst the Shati Community in Jaisalmer (Rajasthan) where the ratio is approximately 550: 1000 (India Tohy), some of the common practices are *dudhapiti* (applying opium on the mother's nipple and feeding the baby), suffocating the girl child with a rug, feeding her poisonous oleander berries, or offering the female baby to the Goddess. This is not to say that mothers do not love their daughters. It is a result of the cultural devaluation of girls. In Bhutan, however, abortions, female infanticide, and child marriages are unheard of (Ministry of Human Resources Development).

Theoretically, the Bhutanese do not discriminate between male and female children. This can be attributed to the Buddhist tradition of non-violence and tolerance, as well as to the Bhutanese system of matrilineal inheritance rights. In contrast to many other South Asian countries, in Bhutan the girl child enjoys a privileged status in a matriarchal society. Marriages are by choice. Divorce and remarriage are easy to arrange and are commonly accepted. Women are actively engaged in production activities, both inside and outside the home. They not only perform agricultural work but also run small shops and businesses. Men, however, still hold all the power in areas related to governance and religion. Similarly, in both the Maldives and Sri Lanka, girls have equal access to life, food, medical care, as well as to love and affection in the family, and educational opportunities.

Education per cent in each age group do not go to school due to the economic problems of low income families. The drop out rate is higher for boys than girls and higher in urban slums, shanties, and remote plantation areas. The gross enrolment ratio has been between 50 to 60 per cent in the South Asian region. While the enrolment of girls has increased in absolute terms, the age group proportionate incidence of drop-outs and stagnation amongst girls has always been higher, especially at the primary level. Furthermore, the rate of non-participation of girls keeps on increasing at the secondary and higher levels. Even in the Maldives, where there is an impressive and almost universal enrolment record at the primary level, empirical evidence suggests a massive drop-out rate right from the primary level (UNICEF, 1989) which increases with every year.

The grim reality is that education up to grade seven is available in the Atolls while higher education is available in the capital, Male. Vocational and employment opportunities for girls are meagre as they do not work in tourist resorts, labour offices, and fisheries, which are the main avenues of employment. The only outlet for adolescent girls is therefore marriage. As a result, girl children in the Maldives experience the same problems of early marriage and too many pregnancies as their Participation of the girl child in educational pursuits, considered to be the most indicative index of human development, has been consistently low in the South Asian region except in Sri Lanka and the Maldives, where there are no educational disparities based on gender, as well as low illiteracy rates of 18.8 and ten per cent respectively (Ministry of Human Resources Development). In Sri Lanka, the family's socio-economic status determines the utilization of resources by boys and girls.

With the introduction of free education from kindergarten to university in 1945, girls have availed themselves of educational opportunities along with the boys, however, eight to ten counterparts in other South Asian countries. Similarly in Bhutan, although there arc equal opportunities for all, parents often question the utility of sending young girls to schools who are expected to perform only household tasks, which they perceive as not requiring schooling or formal education. Moreover, the adolescent girl is a vital support to the family in performing household chores and looking after the elderly as well as younger siblings, even after marriage when she has added responsibilities. In brief, increasing poverty, coupled with a gender bias which compels parents to favour their sons' education over that of their daughters, the high cost of educating girls, conservative cultural values restricting the mobility of adolescent girls the practice of *purdah* in Northwestern Pakistan, rituals associated with menstruation, etc.), the lower number of women teachers, and a constant fear for the safety and chastity of girls have been influencing the participation of girls in educational (both formal and informal) pursuits.

The conflict of the matter is that the curriculum itself, at different levels and in various types of educational programmes in most parts of south Asia, often promotes gender-role stereotyping and instills low self-image among girls. This reinforcement of stereotyped gender roles in the educational system exists in spite of a common core of practical skills being lasted occupations and labour. Never taught in grade six and seven to both boys and girls in Sri Lanka. At the vocational level, girls opt for teaching, nursery, and social work, sewing, tailoring, and home-science courses. As a result they are under-represented in trade and technical courses, which open more remunerative employment avenues for women to realize their full potential.

LABOUR AND EMPLOYMENT

In spite of the general acceptance of the International Labour Organisation (ILO) Convention, child labour is prevalent in this region. According to Swami Agnivesh, child labour flourishes in India even though there is a high level of adult unemployment because it is the cheapest labour available. Statistics of the National Sample Survey revealed that there were 17.58 million girl workers in India in 1985. Non-governmental organizations (NGOS) put this figure at 44.1

million (more than the total population of some of the industrially advanced countries!). A typical female child in the agrarian poor famil'' cooks, cleans, fetches fodder, and water; grazes the cattle, feeds and tends other farm animals; helps in sowing, transplanting, weeding, and harvesting; assists in family based cottage industry; and becomes a surrogate mother to her younger siblings. It is estimated that by the time a girl child reaches the age of 18 years in rural India, she had contributed assistance to the family which is valued at 39,600 rupees (approximately $1300) yet she is perceived as an economic burden.

According to a study in Bangladesh, even very young girls between the ages of seven and nine in large land-owning households work longest of all children: G6 days a year (Palmer). In the urban areas, the girl child performs most of the house- hold and non-household chores, merely replacing agricultural tasks with the requirements most of their work goes unrecognized. Economic pressure and the need for survival compel girls to leave school and work in the formal or informal sectors in countries like Bangladesh, India, and Nepal. They work in unskilled, manual, and low paid jobs in the factories and cottage industries and match industries, fireworks and glass factories, carpet weaving, export-oriented industries, etc.

In the informal sector, they arc employed as maid servants in upper and middle class houses or as rag-pickers. Teenage girls are subjected to exploitation and abuse in the form of lower pay, less security, and excessive occupational health hazards. Carpet weavers, for instance, who are required to sit for long hours every day, develop ankylostomiasis which causes still births and other problems related to child bearing. Many of these girls are sexually exploited by their employers or lured into prostitution. If there is a scarcity of resources, females bear the brunt more than their male counterparts. Needless to say, the arduous work leaves the girl child with less time to dream and less time for play; a denial of her fundamental right to childhood.

MEDIA AND COMMUNICATIONS

Media influences the social ideology. By and large, most media are created by men and women are its recipients. By reinforcing gender stereotypes, systematically glorifying motherhood and subservient wife-hood, the media makes it difficult for adolescent girls in South Asia to bred out of these prescribed roles, norms, and behaviour patterns. The resultant conservative thinking justifies the decision of parents who do not educate their daughters or give them freedom or let them up jobs, and who discriminate between daughters and sons.

GROWTH WITH INEQUALITY

The World Bank claims that poverty in Asia has been halved between 1990 and 2003. But, says John Samuel, the story looks good only until you see the underbelly of this economic growth growing inequality, violence and pollution here's the good news. The economy of Asia is surging ahead. Sustained economic growth seems to have contributed to the reduction of poverty. The World Bank says that poverty rates in Asia as a whole (based on consumption levels of less than $1 per day) have been almost halved in the last decade, falling from 34.3% in 1990 to 19.3% in 2003. Most countries are making steady progress towards achievement of the Millennium Development Goals (MDGs) by 2015.

China, Indonesia, Malaysia, Thailand and Vietnam have all witnessed more than a 50% poverty reduction since 1990 and these countries are supposed to be on track to meet the MDG targets of a further 50% reduction in income poverty by 2015. Literacy rates are going up, infant and maternal mortality is falling, and people are living longer. Asian cities are booming, with signs of prosperity everywhere. More and more billionaires are laughing their way to the banks year after year. The pundits say that the time of Asia has come - it is an Asian Century, with China as the global factory, India as the global office, and the stock exchanges rocking. The story looks good! The story looks good till you notice the underbelly of economic growth: unprecedented levels of inequality, violence, epidemics, congested roads, teeming slums, polluted rivers and failing democracies.

The story looks good till you begin to hear the stories of Dalits, tribals, ethnic minorities, women from the hinterlands of rural deprivation. Stories that you may never read in the newspaper, unheard stories of invisible people, people displaced from land and livelihoods, people who prefer to commit suicide rather than sell their dignity, children who go to bed hungry every single day. Two-thirds of the world's poor live in Asia. There will still be more than a billion people living on less than $ 2 a day in 2015. So is Asia shining? Is economic growth good for billionaires or billons of people? What is the balance sheet of Asia's economic growth? Whose growth is it anyway? Who grows and who loses? Can economic growth alone eliminate poverty in Asia? What are the key challenges for development, democracy and human rights in Asia?

We need to situate the story of economic growth in the well-being, human security and human rights of the most marginalized and excluded people in Asia. In spite of all the growth, if there are still more than one billion people living on less than $2 a day in 2015, the story can turn sour! But it seems the ruling elite and media barons cannot stomach the bad news. Economic growth with inequality creates an economics of deprivation and violence. The present model of economic growth displaces millions of rural and urban poor from their land and livelihoods. As a result of unprecedented displacement due to mining, infrastructure projects and corporate farming, a new generation of social-economic refugees and new poor are emerging across Asia.

They are growing in urban slums, rural areas and in highly concentrated pockets of extreme poverty. A new discontent is brewing and it can adversely affect development, democracy and human rights in Asia. While economic growth helps to create more opportunities for the more educated section of the middle class and a trickle-down effect on a section of the poor, it is creating unprecedented levels of inequality within countries and between countries. Though

China and India, two of the most populous countries in the world, are witnessing high rates of economic growth, there are regions lagging behind in both countries that have poor infrastructure or public service provisions.

The urban and rural poor also face discrimination based on ethnicity, race, religion, caste, gender and place of origin. Women are more marginalized and vulnerable to a system that perpetuates inequality, discrimination and consequent poverty. Economic growth is concentrated in a few urban centres and specially created economically dynamic zones in the costal areas of many countries. But two-thirds of the population in most populous countries like China, India, Indonesia, Bangladesh and Pakistan still lives in rural areas depending on agriculture for their livelihood. Historically marginalized sections like the Dalits in India, ethnic minorities in China and South-East Asia and religious minorities in many countries are alienated from economic growth and the mainstream political process. This urban-centric, uneven and jobless economic growth perpetuates a sort of systemic inequality based on identity, gender and location all over Asia.

Most communities at the receiving end of exclusion are historically marginalized in terms of economic or political opportunities. When inequality has a direct co-relation with identity, it gives rise to new discontents. Such a sense of discontent and shared sense of alienation can often give rise to a new politics of violence reacting to the prosperity of the dominant communities. Surrounding these islands of prosperity is a growing sea of poverty, discontent and consequent reactionary politics. This can perpetuate a cycle of violence, erasing the benefits of growth as well as poverty reduction. So the paradoxical trend of growth with inequality may not be able to sustain growth on a long-term basis. Political stability is a prerequisite for economic growth. Inequality can create more political instability, adversely affecting sustainable economic growth.

This can eventually perpetuate a new cycle of poverty, violence and violation of human rights in Asia. The present economic growth is vulnerable as it is largely dependent on the service sector and the export-oriented manufacturing sector, often at the cost of the agricultural sector that provides livelihoods to the poor and marginalized sections in Asia. This urban-centric growth, with very little investment in rural infrastructure, economy or agricultural, also leads to an unprecedented migration from rural areas to urban areas.

This explosion of populations in urban centres without adequate infrastructure and gainful employment opportunities can create a new generation of urban poor. Urban poverty and inequality with direct links to identity can create more violence against women and escalating crime rates in many countries. Thus the present mode of neo-liberal economic growth is not sustainable in the long run as the billions at the receiving end of marginalization and poverty can spoil the party, giving rise to a new cycle of poverty in Asia.

GENDER AND GLOBALIZATION

"Feminists are always interested in ambivalence", notes Cynthia Enloe in Chapter Fifteen of this outstanding edited collection, "...because so many women live their lives through ambivalence". This powerful statement neatly encapsulates the purpose of the volume, which makes a sustained effort to use work from a variety of disciplines in order to problematize the staid binaries that typically encompass work on gender and globalization. Comprised of eighteen chapters, including an introduction and a conclusion, the book is divided into six thematic areas that provide a basis for the organisation and lines of questioning that shape the authors' arguments: confronting colonial discourses; cultural translations; media; labor, migration and families; trafficking; and militarization. Editors Ferguson and Mironesco specify in their introduction that the work presented throughout the book allows a number of commonalities to emerge "within a dense fabric of specific accounts".

The editors group these common themes into three broad rubrics that run throughout all of the chapters' descriptions of the feminist particularities of place: representations and reproductions; spaces and borders; voices and bodies. Part One, "Confronting Colonial Discourses," is comprised of two chapters. Raiskin notes that Figiel's protagonist, Alofa, is faced with a contradictory set of norms at work in the powerfully gendered institutions of church, family hierarchy and school that organize Samoan adolescent female life.

"While she [Alofa] is taught with violence to suppress her sexual curiosity" Raiskin writes, "the girls [in the novel] are regularly peeped at by neighbors, impregnated by teachers, courted and sometimes raped by male family members... Whom can she [Alofa] believe and what perspective is dictating the conflicting expectations?" Both chapters place a heavy emphasis in their persuasive arguments on the fact that globalization is a manifold process necessarily involving both resistance and accommodation. She notes that while the dissemination of sexually inclusive identities allows right wing conservatives to attribute homosexuality to so-called Western influence, its simultaneous provision of language and a sense of international community "also helps privileged middle-and upper-class gay subjects over a wide range of gendered and sexual subjects in the Indian context".

6

Slum Culture and Social Movements

SOCIAL MOVEMENTS IN THAILAND

Since around 1990, we have seen an outburst of demonstrations, protest marches and new organizations by people of various walks of life. In 1978 there were 42 demonstrations and protests marches, rising to 170 in 1990 and to 988 in 1994. These protests have not been just one-shot events. In most cases participants have organized into a movement to demand their rights, or to fight to protect the environment and their livelihood on a long-term basis.

The sample was not 'representative' in any scientific sense. But it includes many of the most prominent movements, and it indicates something of the variety. This upsurge of political activity cannot be assigned to one group, one grievance, and one cause.

The movements are both varied and complex. Collectively they mark a significant change in our society and politics. The aim of this chapter is to understand something of that change. Let me first summaries the eight studies. Kritiya Atchwanitkul and Kanokwan Tharawan study the movement among women to gain full control over their bodies and sexuality, using four specific cases: the struggle for the rights of women to abort; the campaign for the right to choose a woman as a lover; the women's movements and AIDS; and the fight to eliminate violence against women.

Voravidh Charoenlert deals with women workers' struggle for health and safety in work places. Nalinee Tanthuvanit and Sulaiporn Chonvilai study the roles of poor rural men and women in fights against dam projects which destroyed natural forests and fish breeding grounds and thus took away their means of livelihood, as well as dispersed their communities. Sayamon Kaiyunwong, Atchara Rakyutitham and Krisada Bunchai study the northern hill farmers' movement to win rights to manage local natural resources and to maintain their cultural identities. Praphat Pintoptaeng and Anuson Unno cover the movement by small-scale fishermen in southern Thailand to protect the coastal environment.

Maneerat Mitprasat examines the slum dwellers' movement for housing rights and for participation in urban development. Nualnoi Treerat and Chaiyos Jirapruekpinyo trace the rural doctors' movement against bureaucratic and political corruption in the public health ministry. Narumol Tapchumpon and Charan Ditthapichai focus on the movement for the new constitution of 1997 and the aftermaths. These studies range from the northern hills to the southern coasts, from hill minorities to educated civil servants, from local issues about natural resources to national concerns over constitutional principles.

The nature of the peoples' struggles, their novelty and variety, has motivated this research project. The social movements are not only the expression of discontents of the present; they also represent the collective wishes of large numbers of people. 'Society itself is shaped by the plurality of these struggles and vision of those involved.'

Social movements are controversial. Some political analysts have argued that modern social movements are a dangerous delusion: because these movements emphasize civil society rather than class, networks rather political parties, local action rather than the capture of the state, they result in a futile populist strategy with no hope of success against the entrenched power of the internationalized capitalist state. Defenders have responded that such criticism simply ignores contemporary realities. Class has become much more complex in the globalized, post-industrial world. States are unlikely to be overthrown by old-style movement parties because modern states have impressive resources and broad foundations of tacit support.

Social movements have arisen precisely because of these characteristics of the modern world, and we need to reconcile to these facts rather than cling to an idealized past. Several thinkers have rediscovered the Gramscian discussion of hegemony as a way to reconcile social movements with leftist thinking. Whereas old-style political movements sometimes succeeded in capturing the state, they then often failed to disturb deeper hegemonic ideas such as the domination of one group over another, the exclusion of minorities, the necessity of hierarchy, or the privileges of an elite. Social movements, by contrast, mount direct attacks on such hegemonies from the base of civil society.

Social movements and NGOs have also been criticized, for retarding the development of a political party system which would truly represent the society, and particularly the urban and rural mass. By deflecting people's interest away from the establishment of political parties, these critics suggest, social movements and NGOs cede this realm to old elites and business gangs who directly represent only a minute proportion of the population.

Social movement activists respond that party politics are neither the only type of politics, nor necessarily the most effective for the mass of the people given current structural conditions. In this chapter I first give a brief summary of the worldwide theoretical debate on social movements, which has developed since the 1960s. Then the learning from past debates is analyzed, followed by a discussion of the main features of recent popular movements in Thailand, and ending with a conclusion and dedication.

INTERNATIONAL DEBATES ON SOCIAL MOVEMENTS SINCE THE 1960S

Social movements are simply collective actions - many people acting together. The phrase 'social movement' has taken on new meanings since the 1960s when it was first used to describe anti-war, anti-nuclear, student rights, feminist, gay, and environmentalist movements. Some writers dubbed these campaigns as 'new social movements' because participation cut across class lines and included a large number from the educated white-collar middle class.

The 'new' tag distinguished these movements from movements which were class-based, such as trade unions, communist parties, and socialist movements. The 'social' tag was used because the movements were not directly political. They had no aim to capture or overthrow the state. They tacitly accepted the political framework of liberal democracy. Some wanted to establish different cultural identities, or make the society accept different ways of life (gay, lesbian). Many were about the quality of life, and the assertion of the rights of the individual.

THE US DEBATE

Political scientists argued that these movements demanded new theoretical approaches, different both from the Marxian paradigm of class, and from mainstream theories about interest groups and political recruitment. The first attempts at theorizing in the 1960s and 1970s were in the US. These attempts focused not on why the movements took place (this was seen as being self-evident), but on how they were organized, and why some were more successful than others.

The resource mobilization theory purported to show that the success of a movement depended on the resources available (people, money, allies), and the ability to mobilize these resources (by persuasion, organisation, networking). Resource mobilization theory was wholly about the strategy to make a movement succeed in demanding a change in government policies or legislation. It focused on political action, and paid no attention to civil society.

A variant of this approach became known as political process or political opportunity theory. This approach analyzed the success or failure of movements in terms of the 'opportunities' available. If the government is strong and committed to repression, then the political opportunity is small and the movement likely to fail and *vice versa*. Analysts in this school paid less attention to the 'resources' available, but concentrated on the interaction between the movement on the one hand and the state or other forms of established power on the other.

WESTERN EUROPEAN DEBATE

Debates in Western Europe began a little later than in the US, in the 1970s. From the start, the debates differed from those in the US. This reflected the big difference between the two continents in political history and in the traditions of political theory. The subject of debate was essentially similar - namely new movements about the environment, women and sexual identities. But instead of focusing on strategies and on the requirements for success or failure, the European debate focused on why these non-class-based movements arose.

The early theorists came mostly from Marxist traditions of political economy. They were concerned that Marxist analysis of social movements, which stresses the importance of consciousness, ideology, social struggle and solidarity, seemed inadequate to characterize and explain the new movements. They argued that theories which stress the primacy of structural contradictions, economic classes, and crisis in determining collective identities were inappropriate to understand movements which did not appear to have a class base, and did not seem to be related to any crisis or structural contradiction.

However, the European theorists were not at all impressed by the US theories of resource mobilization and political process. They asserted that present day collective action is not confined to negotiations and strategic calculations to gain political access. Rather, movements involve issues of social norms and identity, and the struggle takes place in the realm of civil society rather than in the realm of politics. The prominent European theorists such as Alain Touraine and Jurgen Habermas linked the upsurge of new social movements to the failure of the democratic system in post-modern society to guarantee individual freedom, equality and fraternity.

In the view of these theorists, the state has become more subject to the market, and democratic processes are being crushed by the growing power of authoritarian technocracy. The power which people once enjoyed through their role in the production process has been eroded by technology and managerial technique. The main socioeconomic role of individuals is not as workers but as consumers, and in this role they are manipulated by the technologies of media and markets. For Touraine, as the technologies of state control, of mega-corporation economics, and of mass communications advance, so the liberty of the individual is diminished.

For Habermas, the expanding structures of state and market economy colonize the public and private sphere of individuals, which he calls the life world. This life world includes the domains in which meaning and value reside - such as family, education, art, religion so private life becomes steadily more politicized by this double encroachment. For Habermas, social movements are defensive reactions to protect the public and the private sphere of individuals against the inroads of the state system and market economy. Similarly, Touraine sees participation in social movements as the only way in which the individual can recover liberty.

For both Habermas and Touraine, the main role of social movements is the mobilization of actors' or 'subjects' - their terms to refer to human beings in their full role as free and creative members of a pluralistic society, as opposed to victims of state and market domination. Social movements in the European theory involve a process of self-awareness to create human and social identities, which are free of the domination of the technocratic state and the market. But the creation of these identities is part of the process of a social movement, not its ultimate goal.

The social movement is a collective form of action to contest the abuses of political and economic power, and to change the political and market institutions in order to produce a better society. Social movements come into conflict with existing norms and values. As put by Cohen and Arato (1992, 511), 'collective actors strive to create group identities within a general identity whose interpretation they contest'. Both the US and Europe are advanced industrial societies with established democratic systems, yet the analysis of social movements in the two continents has differed very widely.

Foweraker explained this difference by reference to the historical context. Western Europe has a history of social democracy, welfare states, institutionalized trade union movements, and strong corporatist traditions linking trade unions with the state. European theorists try to explain the appearance of a new type of social expression by reference to shifts in society and culture. They conclude that the new social movements are concerned with the construction of new social and political identities in opposition to the power of market and state.

In the US by contrast there has been no tradition of social democracy, no trade union corporatism, and no powerful labour movement. Social movements are thus explained not as a consequence of social or structural change, but simply as part of the political manoeuvring whereby groups mobilize resources to gain political representation and to realize social changes. The US theorists are not interested in why social movements arise. They concentrate on why some succeed and some fail.

DEBATES IN LATIN AMERICA

The debate on social movements in the developing world surfaced first in the late 1980s and early 1990s in Latin America

- as a result of the close historical connections between Europe and that region, and because of the heavy American involvement there. Latin American theorists found that many of the insights of the western debate were useful because many movements (women, gay, and environment) were either concerned with similar issues, or were linked in increasingly international arenas of debate.

However, the Latin Americanists also found that local movements, which arose in the region in the 1980s, had many features which required extension or adjustment of the western theories. First, the early movements in Latin America were primarily urban movements resulting from problems of rapid Urbanisation due to industrial development, the capitalization of agriculture, and resulting shifts from rural to urban areas. These urban social movements often revolved around the demand for public utilities, or access to land and water.

The movements gained momentum in part because of the crudeness of the government reaction. Thus the movements themselves were affected by the repressive policies of the state and the suppression of traditional forms of organisation, such as trade unions and political parties. Second, older forms of organisation and agitation such as trade unions and agrarian movements did not disappear. But many new social actors come onto the scene, such as women, teachers, students, ethnic groups, as well as environmental movements.

Third, the movements often involved struggles to establish rights. These included rights to livelihood, rights over the body, rights to land, and 'the right to have rights'. Such movements were not so much expressions of civil society, but rather something much more basic: attempts to create or recover civil society in the face of state power, dictatorial repression, and exclusionary hegemonies. Fourth, these movements were not divorced from the political process, but often by necessity overflowed from civil society into the political realm.

Often movements were locked in contest with authoritarian regimes. As part of their strategy, they demanded democratization, political participation, and constitutional change. While some movements appeared to have the post-modern, non-class-based, networking form of the European model, others were much more obviously class-based and directly political. Fifth, these movements were much more likely than European versions to be concerned with material issues of access to and control over resources such as land, water, and the means of livelihood.

Sixth, while European theory situated new social movements as an extension of the traditions of liberal individualism, many social movements in Latin America were based in communities, leveraged community solidarities, and demanded community rights. Foweraker, for example, studied how the Chiapas movement drew on customary practices within the community as part of network building, and evolved demands for the rights of Mexican Indians as a community. Finally, in Latin America the success rate was not impressive. Repression by the state was tougher and more effective in disrupting and preventing any meaningful success.

Latin American theorists adopted some of the vocabulary and approach of the western literature, but found that they confronted some important differences. At the close of the 1980s, theorists advanced some tentative conclusions. First, they argued that the question of the class base of social movements was an empirical matter. In the advanced world, many movements were either middle-class or cross-class. But in Latin America, most were attempts by the poor and disadvantaged to gain basic rights and improve their economic standing.

Second, they proposed that the success or failure of movements was related not simply to the local strength of the state, but also to the neo-colonial framework and the international backing for local state power. Touraine's observations about the domination of state system, market economics, and mass communications had to be modified to stress the extreme nature of this domination in the situation where the power-base of state, market, and communication media was remote from the local context and hence even more difficult to oppose.

In the early 1990s, two new developments in the Latin American movements prompted still further extension and adaptation of social movement theory. The first development was a much larger prominence of rural social movements, with the spread of land-grab movements and the explosion of the Chiapas peasant resistance. The second was the paradoxical development in the political economy, which saw a revival of democratic forms of government running in parallel with rapid widening of the gaps between rich and poor, powerful and powerless.

The explosion of rural movements further emphasized the importance of competition over resources. It also drew the focus back to issues of identity, culture, and community. Many of the movements in Latin America were centred among minority groups, which drew some of their movement's strength from reassertion of identity. Even in cases where ethnicity was not such an explicit issue, movements drew on a background of rural identity and culture raised in opposition to a dominant urban ideology of market and state.

Similarly, movements drew on concepts of community, which found little place in the theories worked out within the liberal-individualist traditions of the west. The paradox of democracy and social division drew attention to the special conditions of subordinate societies within an increasingly globalized world. Latin American theorists argued that the region's urban centres and urban elites were being annexed (politically, economically and culturally) to a globalized world system dominated by the USA.

In this process, the power of the national state was diminished. Hence, even though dictatorships were being replaced by democratic politics, there was no space for meaningful negotiation of social and economic demands. The strength of internationally backed repression meant that local political defiance was increasingly ineffective. The decline of trade unions and welfare provisions was evidence of this trend.

Hence social movements acquired a new importance as a basis for defiance.

DEBATES IN INDIA

In the 1980s, the debate spread more widely in the developing world. In India there was a long tradition of socialist and communist movements prior to the 1980s. The social movements in the 1980s took on new features in several respects. To begin with, many old causes declined in importance. The trade union movement, for example, had previously campaigned heavily for nationalization of industries or for increasing the state's role in managing privately owned industrial enterprises. Over the 1980s, this issue disappeared. Similarly, the movement for land reforms - in the sense of reallocating land from big landlords to the landless - diminished in importance.

At the same time, movements related to community, minorities, religion, women's rights, natural resources and the environment grew in importance. Untouchables demanded that the government increase their quota of civil service posts. Environmental movements protested against big dam projects and demanded alternative development strategies. Local communities demanded rights to manage local resources. Small farmers demanded specific forms of government support. None of these new movements adhered to the old socialist ideology and none seemed to have a definite idea of an 'ideal society'.

According to Omvedt, the social movements in India in the 1980s differed significantly from those occurring previously. The participants showed no interest in class analysis, but insisted on the specific nature of the exploitation they suffered. They were unimpressed by socialist ideology as a way to explain their position. They rejected alignment with leftist political organisation as a strategy for redress. Omvedt concluded that these new movements in India required researchers and analysts to re-imagine the whole of the Indian society.

The varied movements expressed a new cultural dynamism. Although the individual movements were scattered and diverse, together they amounted to a rejection of old ideologies and values, namely the dominant high-caste Brahmanism, the state system constructed since independence, and the integration of Indian society into post-cold war global capitalism. The aim of the movements was to find new ways to affect change. Orthodox Marxists reacted strongly against Omvedt's analysis.

Utsa Patnaik argued that the emphasis on culture and identity were signs of backwardness and anti-modernism. Brass (1994) argued that the new movements were suffused by various forms of false consciousness (post-modernism, communitarianism), and were a threat to the traditions of socialist political organisation. But Omvedt countered that leftists had to accept the new movements for what they were, rather than arguing that they should be something different. She urged theorists to analyze new social movements in order to adapt old ideas of class analysis and political mobilization to fit with the new reality. In her view there must be a reinterpretation of revolution.

LEARNING FROM PAST DEBATES

Two things emerge from the above discussion. First, the movements, which emerged in Thailand in the 1990s, have many similarities to the Latin American and Indian cases. Second, the theorists in Latin America and India found many useful elements in the studies of social movements in the west, but also found many differences in their local situations. Before turning to the Thai experience, let us summarize four key areas where the Latin American/Indian debates have modified or rejected the western models.

DOUBLE DOMINATION

Touraine (and other European theorists) argue that new social movements are specific to a post-modern society - by which he means a society in which the major part of the workforce are educated, skilled, white-collar, and probably in service industries. However, the technocratic states, market forces, and mass communications which Touraine identifies as the forces oppressing humanity and making social movements necessary, are clearly present in societies which cannot yet be called post-modern. Indeed, this domination is a global process.

Hence the diminution of liberty, which this dominance entails is also present in non-western societies, and also needs to be opposed. Indeed, many of the new movements in the non-western world have been focused precisely against the power of the state, the expansion of big business at the expense of small, and the monopolies over modern communications. But the problems have become more complicated in non-western countries by the extra dimension of subordination or dependency to a western dominated world. The dominating forces, which Touraine identifies, are globalized. The big businesses are multinational.

The mass communication systems are US-owned and global in scope. National state systems are being weakened and co-opted. Touraine talks about social movements contesting directly against corporate and state power. In non-western countries, the contest is more complex because these powerful forces are more remote, and the balance of power even more unequal. Social movements in developing countries must be seen in the context of a double repression: at the local level by the power structure of the society and the market forces in question; and at another global level by the forces of world capitalism and multinational corporations.

SOCIAL OR POLITICAL

Theories constructed for the west are concerned with movements, which focus on the quality of life, rather than on the material aspects of life. The movements' actors are often those in the middle class. In non-western countries, where the material aspects are still a problem, many social movements are about bread and butter issues, particularly access to resources. The actors involved in many cases are the underprivileged, the marginalized, workers, and poor farmers.

In a sense, Latin America and other similar parts of the world are experiencing at the same time two different types of movement which in the western case took place in two historically separate phases. Moreover, these two types cannot be simply separated. Because they exist in the same place and time, they are inevitably interrelated - through people, organizations, network, shared context. Two important features of the recent movements in the developing world have been struggles for livelihood, and demands for basic rights.

In most cases, the struggles are by definition political, because they have to challenge the political control of resources, and the political arrangements for the allocation of rights. Hence, it is questionable how far these movements deserve to be labelled 'social', in the sense that this suggests they are not 'political'. And it is questionable how far they deserve to be labelled 'new' when much of their content is very traditional. Because of this, the use of the term 'new social movement' has declined in use, and been replaced by 'popular movement'.

FROM DEMOCRACY TO PEOPLE POLITICS

Many of the movements in developing countries since the 1980s aimed to establish or strengthen democratic systems and structures, in the belief that this was an important precondition for removing oppression, allowing participation, and hence overcoming many of the inequalities and injustices in the society and economy. But recent experience suggests that this democratizing goal is important but insufficient. States have retained their authoritarian character even while taking on many of the outward forms of democracy. They have access to modern technology and communications of social control. Their authoritarianism is sometimes reinforced by global forces.

The theoretical equality under a democratic system is ineffective when there are large differences in income leading to 'money politics'. In these circumstances, democratization is ineffective in challenging economic inequalities or embedded social hierarchies. Hence there has been a shift away from democratization to 'people politics', which implies more direct participation of people in the decision making process on matters which affect their livelihoods and their ways of life.

INDIVIDUAL AND COMMUNITY

Touraine, and other western thinkers are writing firmly in the historical traditions of western liberalism with its emphasis on individualism. Touraine is explicit in wanting to revive the ideals of the French Revolution with its emphasis on liberty, equality, fraternity - especially on liberty. However, in the non-western world, which has a different historical tradition and a much shallower experience of advanced capitalism, such an emphasis on individual liberty is either absent or much weaker.

Often it is an importation with uncertain local roots. Local traditions of philosophy and political practice place more emphasis on the role of communities and groups. Touraine has to go through some complex argument to explain why a social movement (which involves collective actions) is a way for an individual to reclaim liberty. In the non-western context, this stage of the theorizing can be (and often already is) conveniently by-passed. Communities are resurrected, reinvented or re-imagined as the basis of new movements of defiance against the power of state and markets, as well as the guide for alternative development of a desirable future society.

Many social movements in the developing world since the 1970s have been based in poor, peripheral, or minority communities. The Chiapas movement is a classic case in point. In Thailand the farmers movements (the Assembly of the Poor, the small fishermen's and the northern hill farmers' movements) all have a base in the community, or are community movements, not individual movements. Chairat (2538) has analyzed the discourse on community culture as a social movement based in the village community.

These movements have pressed for alternative development strategies, or imagined ideal future societies, different from those of the ruling mainstream. Sometimes they have sought to protect community rights against the inroads of market individualism. Sometimes they have actively revived community solidarity and community cultures as political strategy. Sometimes they have demanded that the broader society accepts and respects the culture and values of a minority or repressed community.

In sum, while European theory describes movements which operate in civil society, reject old forms of political organisation, challenge post-modern forces of state and market, and seek to defend traditions of liberal individualism, those that have appeared in the non-western world seem to be very different. They are often movements of the poor and oppressed. They cannot avoid confronting the political structure. They are increasingly involved in combating forces of globalization. They are often based in the community and draw on its strengths.

RECENT POPULAR MOVEMENTS IN THAILAND

The upsurge of popular movements in Thailand over the past decade obviously shares many similarities with the experience of Latin America and India - the broad base of participation; rejection of old forms of organisation, emphasis on environment, and role of community discourse. But there are certain ways in which the details or emphasis of the movements in Thailand have been importantly different.

HISTORICAL SHIFT

A large number of movements of great variety have arisen within a very short space of time. In a broad sense, this is a result of changes in the global and local context. The end of the cold war has led to the decline of dictatorship. The opening up of democratic politics has created more space for social agitation and political expression. The global discourse on topics such as rights, identity, and environmental protection has stimulated reactions within Thailand. At the same time, the rise of the modern state, market-oriented economy, and new forms of global power (hegemonic states, and dominant multinationals) has caused conflicts over resources, dislocation of communities, and erosion of ways of life. In sum, the combined impact of democratization, economic growth, and globalization creates contradictory results. They encroach on people's lives and livelihood, and at the same time they open up political opportunities and give legitimacy to social movements.

The new movements in Thailand include a wide variety of social groups. But the significant fact is the large participation by the 'little people' who have traditionally been excluded from a political voice. These include hill peoples, small fishermen, marginal peasants, slum dwellers, and working women. They have become more assertive than before about their rights and roles in society. This is partly explained by the passing of the Cold War and the era of dictatorial rules. But there has also been an important synergy between these various different movements. The space created by one movement is available to another. Experiences feed on one another and become cumulative.

The sum of several movements is greater than their individual contributions alone. This upsurge is significant because it represents a break from the past. Thai society has had little or no experience of mass political mobilization. Nationalism was orchestrated by the elite. With no colonial control, there was no anti-colonialist mass movement. Socialism was crushed within the context of the cold war. Hence the social movements of the 1990s represent some of the first, sustained examples of mass social action. With an ever faster pace of globalization, social movements are definitely here to stay in Thailand.

DEMOCRATIC LIMITS

In different ways, various movements express frustration over the poor operation of Thailand's parliamentary democracy. The rapid rise of 'money politics' has stimulated middle class support for the movement for constitutional reform and campaigns against corruption such as that in the public health ministry. The failure of representative democracy to provide any meaningful representation for poor and marginal groups has stimulated many agitational campaigns. Despite wide differences in social background, these various movements share a feeling that politicians and bureaucrats imagine themselves as a ruling caste rather than as public servants.

This shared perspective can at times become a basis for common action. The Assembly of the Poor supported the constitutional movement although the constitution was peripheral to their major concerns. Many of the activists in campaigns over the constitution and corruption have lent moral and organizational support to little people's campaigns for rights and resources. Of course, such cooperation has strict limits. But in the short term it helps to create a 'snowball' effect of benefit to many contemporary movements.

Environment

Over half the movements covered in the project are concerned in some way with the environment and competition over natural resources. Over the past half century, natural resources have been captured and destroyed for private gain, with the process often justified by discourses about development and national interest. Those most sensitive to the loss of such resources are the little people who depend most heavily on nature for their livelihood and culture. The attempts to halt this process aswhich transcends any particular local campaign, and acts as a common base for alliance between groups of varying background.

The past pattern of development assumed that lots of little people could be sacrificed in the business of creating modern industrial society on the model from the west. But the recent movements show that it has become more difficult to maintain that belief. The government will have to think more seriously in pursuing old policies and strategies without regards to the effects on people and to their wishes.

Women

One striking feature of this upsurge of popular movements has been the role of women. This includes involvement in movements on specifically female issues (such as those studied by Kritaya), but also a leading role in other campaigns. Women have been a major force in the labour movement (Voravidh), in slum campaigns (Maneerat), in rural protests (Nalini), and in the constitutional campaign (Naruemon). This is significant because it offers a strong contrast to the extreme male bias in Thailand's formal public life.

The female share among parliamentarians, senior bureaucrats, and local politicians is very small. Traditionally women had a strong role in Thai society. In the realms of the family and local community, there have never been traditions of suppressing the female contribution. The male bias in formal politics developed within the modern bureaucracy and political system based on western models. The strong and often leading roles taken by women in modern popular movements represent a reassertion of traditional female power.

CULTURE, IDENTITY, ALLIANCE

As in other developing countries Thai social movements mobilize concepts of culture and identity to build solidarity and inspire action. This is similar to earlier western movements, but also importantly different. The cultures and identities mobilized are very often those of the poor, the peripheral, and the excluded. This gives these movements some of the moral power (against injustice) of old-style class-based action.

But at the same time, the fact that these movements are not founded explicitly on class concepts and motivated by class antagonism makes it easier for them to mobilize support from a broader public. Appeals to universally acceptable concepts - protection of the environment, health for all, no corruption -

make it possible for movements of the underprivileged to build support from the educated middle class, through the links forged by NGOs.

NGO's

Around the world, the role of NGOs has become controversial. To what extent do they actually create the movements, which they claim only to facilitate? What is the moral or political justification for their role? Are they a force for democracy, or are they helping destroy democracy by diverting attention from parties, parliaments, and other official democratic institutions? Are they part of the globalizing forces which are undermining sovereignty and national government? Our study did not set out to be an in-depth study of the role of NGOs. But the above questions are so much part of current debate that it is worth offering some tentative conclusions which arise from the project.

In terms of its resource base, the Thai NGO movement remains rather weak. The numbers of people directly involved on a full-time basis are small. Funding is very limited. Foreign funds and assistance are available and important, but they are not large. At the same time, NGOs have played an important role in all of the movements studied in the project. It is probably fair to say that without the NGO contribution, several of these movements would be significantly weaker and less effective. What then explains the fact that the NGO movement is weak in resources but able to exert such an impact? In part this is simply due to the levels of effort and commitment on the part of a small number of people. But there are also structural and strategic aspects.

The roles which the NGO workers play are very specific. They accumulate practical political experience which allows them to serve as effective advisors on strategy and tactics. They act as transmitters of information between groups and across movements, which allows local groups to shorten the learning curve. They have contact networks which can bring in expertise (from international sources, academics, researchers), and which can pass out publicity to the press and other media. They have educated skills which are important for compiling documents, conducting negotiations, framing publicity, and so on. In none of these roles do the NGOs have the ability to create movements, though they certainly can contribute to making them stronger. The NGO workers themselves argue that whatever role they have is dependent on the strength of the popular movement which they assist.

This NGO role has arisen because of the upsurge of popular movements on the one hand, and on the other, the authorities' attempt to combat these movements by a mixture of constructive neglect or the exercise of traditional power. Often the NGOs are described as a 'middle class' element. As a recent study has shown, many of the older (1970s) generation of Thai NGOs did have middle class backgrounds, and were motivated by political commitment; however, those of the new generation (1990s) are more likely to come from a rural or urban lower-class family, to have climbed the ladder of educational achievement, and to have made a decision to remain true to their roots.

Strategies

Among those in Thailand committed to social and political change, three general strategies for action are being debated. The first is to work within the existing system and to press for changes in law, law enforcement, institutions, and mindsets, through various forms of social action and political lobbying. The second alternative is to form a political party to provide a more direct channel for change. The third alternative is the so-called New Anarchism - people should just ignore the state, pursue their preferred way of life, and seek strength within the community and through networking between communities.

Most popular movements in Thailand adopt the first option. The anarchist solution is problematic because of the intrusive power of the state (particularly in control over natural resources), and because of the difficulty of evading various forms of hegemony handed down from history. The option of establishing a new political party has been actively debated in recent years, but to date most activists fear that the result would be infighting, disunity, and distraction from the goals of direct social action and counter-hegemonic political activism.

The project on the social movements, upon which this chapter is based, was an academic research project, but it was also conceived as a contribution to the movements being studied. All of the principal researchers and their assistants working on the eight case studies were chosen because they are committed activists. I hoped they would profit in some way by being asked to research these movements and reflect on the forces behind them, the strategies adopted, the successes, and the failures. That much was intentional. But beyond that, the subjects of the research got involved in the project in ways that I had not expected. In an early work-in-progress seminar, an activist was orchestrating the fishermen's blockade of Phangnga bay over his mobile phone from the back of the room.

At the final seminar in October 2000, several of the dam protesters attended and cheered on the researcher. Leaders of the doctors' movement came to the presentation on the public health scandal, contributed advice and information, and insisted on presenting a garland to the research team. And one man from the Hmong hill community attended the seminar to get tips on how to help his home village, which had been ransacked by vigilantes egged on by the forest department a few days earlier. One of the important aspects of modern popular movements is that they are not confined within any formal frame.

ASIAN CITIES AND CULTURAL CHANGE

The past twenty years have witnessed the decisive end of attempts at state-centred urban planning in Mumbai. The post-Independence Development Plan, which has guided land, housing, and economic growth since the sixties, has been displaced in favour of piecemeal investments in infrastructure and transport, and housing and slum rehabilitation by the state, with increased participation from private builders and agencies. With the retreat of the state from its ambitious agendas of rational land-use, equitable distribution of services and resources, and protection of the environment, the instruments of abstract spatial planning used by the state have withered and mutated into new urban forms marked by severe exclusions and enclosures. Classical urban planning practice was historically premised on the segregation of the functions of modern urban life into residential, commercial/industrial, and public spheres, and their centralized location governed by state directives.

However, Asian cities have constantly demonstrate the falsity of this separation of functions - with their vast districts of dense, mixed-use settlements governed by porous legalities, popular politics, and tactical negotiations over space and survival. This vast and complex economy has been inadequately imagined as the Third World 'slum' or theorized as the 'informal economy'. With the retreat of the state, centralized planning practice and its technocratic spatial imagination has been appropriated into a new spatial regime in which a predatory class of private builders dominates the production of formal housing for a minority of the rich, amidst rising inequality in access to housing and basic services for the majority of the urban poor in Mumbai.

Modern, western approaches to architecture, urban design and planning still treat urban housing as a place of residence, domesticity, and leisure as a privileged site of social relations, and a prized object of consumption. However, a greater understanding of the cultural history of Asian cities must situate urban housing as a key unit of production in the urban economy, the material grid and medium through which everyday politics and culture are experienced. In mega-cities like Mumbai, the dissolution of large manufacturing industries in the eighties, and growth of new elite-oriented service economies in the nineties, has elevated the construction industry and land speculation into the primary circuits of cash and capital accumulation in the city.

While a functional and economic separation of home and workplace is a central tenet of modern urban spatial practice, in Asian cities like Mumbai this false spatial division poses severe obstacles to situating the production of housing as part of the larger 'informal' economy of small scale manufacturing, casual labour, and flexible employment which defines the urban landscape for the majority of the urban poor. Such a classical understanding of the role of the housing economy also lends support to the predatory urbanism and its regime of speculative accumulation, legal exclusion, and the violence of mass demolitions of the homes and workshops of the urban poor.

The valorization of the middle-class home and over-consumption in the urban media has its parallel in the marginalization of the majority of the urban poor from land and housing - some 60% of the urban population of around 14 million citizens. Secure housing is now the most desired object of consumption by all classes, from land-less squatters and working slum-dwellers to established tenants and the middle classes. The new social and spatial relations of global Mumbai have given rise to various movements for housing and tenancy rights, and are now becoming the main arena for public politics.

Our presentation will focus on two practical interventions by the Collective Research Initiatives Trust (CRIT) in these new urban landscapes in Mumbai, on understanding urban housing as social practice in the contemporary city. The first interventions include an online platform, called the Mumbai Free Map, in which a digital base map of Greater Mumbai is being made available in an accessible and interactive web-based interface. Through this platform built completely on open source software, copy left city maps, and public geo-data communities can read and write free information on their neighbourhoods, buildings, public spaces and environment and assess the existing opportunities for self-development. This information, while ostensibly 'public', has previously only available to a closed circuit of builders, municipal officials, and their agents, and our hope is to create a new medium for communities to realize their spatial rights in Mumbai.

The second intervention by CRIT which we shall discuss is a programme for Community Housing Support providing financial models, policy advice, and architectural, design and information services to urban poor communities seeking to redevelop their housing through an open and decentralized design and financial model, with communities replacing builders as the agents of self-development. In this programme, CRIT is working with local housing associations in the Mumbai Tenants Federation and Slum Rehabilitation Society.

Through an open design and production process, communities are actively involved in the design and construction of integrated home and work units, spatial types which allow for inclusion and flexibility. The model of developing a community corpus to finance the housing project also allows use of the often lucrative profits from commercial land values to be reinvested in the maintenance of the housing by the community as a secure asset. The presentation will focus on the new geographies of community resistance to the predatory forces of the new metropolitan environment, through our work with local housing rights movements and associations of the urban poor.

While the Asian city is famous for its rich local geographies and exotic cultural mixes, we need more detailed studies and analyses of the cultural history of housing in Asian cities - both as a material technology and as a social practice. The tactics and negotiations of urban poor communities in the context of Mumbai's contemporary housing crisis indicate a new form of urban politics. The future directions will be articulated by a historical understanding of the production of urban housing as material culture in the Asia Pacific.

7

Slum Culture in Daily Life

THE URBANISATION OF POVERTY

In the past fifty years, the Philippines have experienced what can be called "the Urbanisation of poverty." This process describes the shift in the concentration of poor people from the village to the city, bringing about various social problems, such as massive unemployment and the proliferation of slums. Beyond the movement of poor people, this concept pertains to the various historical and social factors that have led to the poverty of many urban dwellers. However, the Urbanisation of poverty can also be viewed alternatively as the "poverty of Urbanisation," which points to the limitations of our understanding of urbanity and its many consequences. This conceptual weakness often results in poor urban plans and urban development strategies, eventually causing the failure of the urban system to create a better living environment and provide for the needs of most people.

URBANISATION AND POVERTY IN THE PHILIPPINES

The Philippines urbanized rapidly from 1960 to 1990, during which the urban population increased its share of the total population from 29.8 percent to 48.8 percent. Toward the mid-1990s, studies indicated that the percentage of people in urban areas was already at 50 percent. Recent census reports, though, showed that the figure decreased to 48.05 percent in the second half of the 1990s. This change can be attributed to three major factors. First is the saturation of urban space that inhibits its capacity to accommodate more migrants from rural areas. Second is the implementation of countryside development programmes, such as agriculture and fishery, and peripheral industrialization, such as the establishment of export processing zones, that must have held people from moving to urban centers, or attracted skilled urban dwellers to move to these new "growth areas."

The third is the migration of skilled urban residents overseas. Although these data imply that the Philippines are not yet a predominantly urbanized society, it does not necessarily mean that there are less people in urban areas. Despite the disruption of the expected urban-rural population distribution trend, the number of urban residents still rose from 29.64 million in 1990 to 36.76 million in 2000 (NSO 2000). Clearly, congestion and poverty in many urban areas remain among the major problems in the country. The growth of the urban population, increase in poverty incidence, and consequent proliferation of informal settlements are often associated with the massive migration of rural residents to urban centers, especially to Metro Manila.

Despite government efforts to curtail their growth, the rural migrant population has increased steadily in recent decades owing to the declining agricultural production in the countryside and the continuing peace and order problems in some rural areas. When rural people come to the cities, they seek out places that can help maximize their limited resources, such as areas where housing is inexpensive and where relatives and town mates are close by to provide them with the orientation and social capital necessary to survive in the urban jungle. They choose to live with people who understand their way of life and who had migrated to the city for the same reason as theirs. What the migrants do not seek and do not foresee are the permanency and the deterioration of these settlements.

In most cases, people move to slum areas that deteriorate further as more poverty-stricken migrants continue to arrive. Natural growth also contributes to the increasing number of people in urban areas. Many informal settlers are second- or third-generation migrants. Given that efforts to address the problems of informal settlers are limited, poverty is passed on from one generation to the next, like inheritance. With this condition, the phenomenon of urban poverty in the Philippines has continued to grow at alarming proportions. As of 2002, the urban poor had comprised 55 percent of the total poor population in the country, and some 1.4 million households lived in informal settlements.

URBAN DEVELOPMENT AND THE STATE IN THE PHILIPPINES

The Philippine government is confronted with major challenges posed by the growth of urban poor communities, especially as land, basic services, and livelihood opportunities are becoming less sufficient. Various administrations have sought to address the illegal occupation of land by the urban poor. In the 1960s, the government's strategies largely involved relocation and on-site development through the provision of housing and opportunities for land acquisition. Many of these initiatives failed to fulfill the needs of their target beneficiaries. Relocation sites were far from clustered commercial areas where people could obtain employment, and lacked the basic services that would have encouraged the people to stay.

Government also discounted the importance of providing the beneficiaries of its low-cost housing projects with livelihood opportunities to enable them to support their basic daily needs, as well as to pay the amortization of their acquired housing units. In many cases, beneficiaries were forced to sell their land and houses to generate money, and ended up returning to the city, more often, to squat again. Meanwhile, on-site development could accommodate only a small number of people because of limited budget and space. Funds allocated for housing were low, as housing did not figure among the priorities of government.

Fewer land parcels were available, since public real estate properties had already been used for infrastructure and other facilities. Private landowners often disapproved plans to use their properties for socialized housing. Government-funded housing projects, such as the Philippine Homesite and Housing Corporation and the Bagong Lipunan Improvement of Sites and Settlements (BLISS), and indirect provident fund schemes, such as Pag-IBIG, had had negligible impact on overall housing provision because these generally favored middle- income groups, especially government employees.

Demolitions of informal settlements to make way for the construction of various infrastructure projects became a regular occurrence from the late 1950s to the early 1980s. In some cases, the affected communities were not provided with relocation sites or an assurance of slots in government housing projects. The threat of displacement by these demolitions drew the informal settlers together. Confrontations between government forces that were often composed of military or police personnel and the residents often resulted in violence. In the past thirty years, however, the informal settlers have grown in strength and number owing to the advocacy and organizing efforts of the academic, religious, labor, and non-government organizations. They have become aware of their rights to decent housing and begun to assert their demands in urban development plans.

Many of the recent attempts to demolish informal settlements had been futile, as the residents insisted on staying on their lots, being granted the necessary tenure rights, and being provided with the basic infrastructure and services enjoyed by the rest of the city. They have increasingly fought for their stake in the land they have occupied for several years, and no longer easily submit to offers of relocation or socialized housing. The growth of local organizations and government's realization of the difficulties in providing housing to its growing urban poor population have led to a radical change in government's mass housing policy. Beginning in the mid-1970s, government paid attention to slum upgrading - the observance of the maximum retention policy in informal settlements - as an alternative to the resettlement or relocation programme.

After the 1986 "People Power" Revolution, socialized housing policies have shifted from the state-centered development approach to a people-centered and aided self-help approach. In this strategy, the role of the state is changed from that of provider to facilitator as a way of bringing the nongovernment sectors to the provision of housing and utilizing their creative capacities and resources.

The Research Problem

Slum upgrading offers the best framework for addressing urban poverty because it presents the most comprehensive strategy that can deal with the various aspects of the problem. Aside from providing decent housing and access to land, slum upgrading can integrate and address other important urban poor issues, such as micro enterprise development and the provision of basic services. Given the various weaknesses of slum upgrading, however, a better understanding of the factors facilitating and inhibiting its scaling up has been identified as critical in addressing the continually expanding problem of urban poverty. As slum upgrading has been widely accepted, looking at the experiences and innovative upgrading practices of certain communities can generate important lessons for more effective urban development and poverty alleviation initiatives.

In pursuing this interest, the following questions are of interest:

1. How does slum upgrading influence the development of a locality?
2. How do people respond to the opportunities and challenges posed by slum upgrading initiatives?

Slum Upgrading as a Social Process

The slum upgrading that has been implemented in the past fifteen years in Barangay Commonwealth is rather difficult to operationalize, and even much more difficult to quantify. It is almost impossible to effectively isolate the improvements to a specific time, event, or setting, since most of the projects happen spontaneously and many are still ongoing. What can be traced is the beginning of the upgrade; the end is something that the barangay always has to catch up to - a state that seems unattainable but has to be accomplished. Not that the upgrading has always been short-handed; rather, different issues and challenges can always surface as localities continue to develop. Slum upgrading in Barangay Commonwealth has involved an unending process of negotiation, a series of bargaining, dealings, and compromises by the different stakeholders.

Key Indicators of Slum Upgrading

Several key indicators can be given serious consideration in examining slum upgrading initiatives in the NGC, where Barangay Commonwealth is located. These are (1) land security; (2) improvement in the socioeconomic conditions of residents; (3) opportunities for participation and self-determination; and (4) provision of basic services. These key indicators may be provided or brought about by government, the local organizations, or a partnership between the two or with other actors. First, security of tenure is believed to be the most important indicator of an upgrade. Although a land title, as some would say, is "just a piece of paper," its value goes beyond the entitlement that legitimizes the use and appropriation of the real property by its legal owner. Security of tenure also determines the capacity of an individual to improve his or her property.

For instance, the city hall issues building permits only if the property on which the structure will be built has a legal land title. Likewise, landownership can motivate people to develop their property since they can reap its long- term benefits. When people have no security of tenure, they will always feel threatened by demolitions and the consequent loss of investment in the land. In Barangay Commonwealth, those who have permanent and improved houses are generally those who have acquired land titles as beneficiaries of housing projects. Second, if one owns land but does not have the means to maintain it, build a house on it, or utilize it for economic gain, the property is worth only its computed market value, but not its use in providing shelter or improving people's lives, which is the end goal of urban slum upgrading.

A permanent job or a means of livelihood is necessary for one to provide his or her family with a decent life. It also signifies an opportunity for advancement in the future. Third, it is highly accepted that the sustainability of a development intervention can be assured only if certain institutional mechanisms are in place at the local level to continue the activities after the formal programme is completed. This institutional mechanism, however, requires that people participate in and have a "sense of ownership" of the project.

This helps prevent alienation among the local people, who usually feel that their lives are being controlled by external agents, such as community organizers or project officers. Instead, this assures that people are aware that the project is theirs, and that their actions will determine the kind of future they will have. Local participation can also enable the slum upgrading programme to capitalize on the people's creative capacities and resources.

Lastly, upgrade does not just about own the land; fulfilling one's basic needs is just as essential an indicator. In informal settlements, families require support services, such as medical care and education, to maintain a generally acceptable living condition. The presence of these forms of assistance will motivate them to participate in processes that will allow the locality to sustain the level of upgrade it has achieved. A more important question is: Why does slum upgrading seem to follow a process of perpetual transition?

Culture of Improvisation

People's response to slum upgrading is characterized by patterns of coping strategies evident in how they generally deal with the compound conditions of poverty. The uncertainties that the urban poor face force them to "improvise" in order to survive in a fast-changing world that is increasingly making their lives more difficult. Because of limited resources and the various conditions that shroud their capacity to take hold of their future, the urban poor come up with short-term, quick-fix solutions to each problem as it arises. These coping strategies become part of the people's culture and turn into a stock of knowledge which supplies people with interpretations and guides of action as they confront opportunities and challenges in their lives.

Perhaps no other place in the world is more frequently devastated by calamities and disasters than the Philippines. Its location within the "typhoon belt" and "the ring of fire" often puts the country at the whipping end of nature's wrath. Having to cope with this hard reality, Filipinos have learned to be resilient, resourceful, and innovative in order to survive difficult situations. For instance, given the fact that what one has built for years can be easily destroyed in one night, the early ancestors of the Filipinos never erected permanent residential structures, which were common to other ancient civilizations. What is the use of building stone structures when a single jolt of a strong earthquake can topple everything to the ground? Instead, structures were constructed to be adaptable, something that could be built and rebuilt in a short period of time.

Houses were usually made from simple materials that were readily available and could be easily processed. These had to be built quickly to avoid the next rainy season. Besides, a long duration of construction was not advisable since it could be interrupted by an unexpected typhoon. In case of damage, these structures were repaired immediately so that these could be useful again. The storm-battered Ivatan of Batanes Islands, for instance, lived in simple timber-and-thatch houses until the Spanish taught them how to build their famous *chivuvuhong* and *sinarampadan* (stone houses). Understanding the reality of creation and destruction as part of everyday life, Filipinos have developed the "culture of improvisation," a way of life that is characterized by adaptation, creativity, and innovation.

A quintessential example of this culture of improvisation is the *bahay kubo* (nipa hut). Geography and climate, the available natural building materials, and local construction skills influenced the design and construction of the *bahay kubo*. Aside from the ingenuity in the use of local materials, the *bahay kubo* is appreciated for its functionality. Its thick roof of thatch insulates the interior from the tropical sun; rain slides down its steep roof, and wide overhangs protect the walls from water; the floor of bamboo slats conducts air into the house even if all openings are shut. However, the *bahay kubo* is also known as the dwelling of the peasant, the longstanding epitome of poverty in the Philippines. Hence, it is held as a symbol of material impoverishment, especially when seen alongside the *bahay na bato* (stone houses) of the rural elite.

So when peasants move to the city, they bring with them their ability to make use of whatever is available. In adapting to a new setting, the peasant becomes the urban poor and the *bahay kubo* evolves into the *barong-barong* (shanty). Just like its rural predecessor, the barong-barong is constructed from whatever materials that the urban poor can salvage from their immediate environment. And like the *bahay kubo*, the barong-barong is generally built with a degree of speed. This is not only to avoid unfavorable weather but also to evade landowners and authorities. And rebuilding the barong-barong is just as easy once it is damaged by natural calamities or, in many cases, destroyed by demolition drives.

This is why in many instances; new structures sprout a few hours after the demolition crew leaves. This culture of improvisation also applies when looking at the layout of the entire shantytown. Because of their dubious beginnings, the existence of informal settlements seems to be always shrouded in contrived obscurity. Informal settlements are often like "nowhere places," residents have no clear addresses, streets are not well arranged, and the entrance to these localities often involves climbing walls or walking along a narrow creek embankment. Having no legitimate existence, these localities are often referred to by people according to "real places" (e.g., Alabang Gillage [beside a village], home along the riles [railroad track]) in establishing their locations.

However, this obscurity is not only a result of geographical displacement but also a form of improvisation by the people to protect their localities against authorities as well as to assert their claim to a particular space in the city amidst the many threats and various forms of exclusion. During the early period of settlement in Barangay Commonwealth, for instance, some relatively more well-off settlers did not build their houses from concrete and made these look like shanties to hide the fact that some settlers were not really that poor. Even slum upgrading, which was designed originally as a permanent solution, has become a series of temporary responses to a continually evolving issue of urban poverty in the Philippines - a series of improvisations rather than a complete solution. In fact, most forms of intervention in slum upgrading programmes have tended to be reactive and situational.

Problems are often addressed only when they arise, and some site-specific strategies are difficult to apply in other areas. Hence, it is difficult to conceptualize slum upgrading in the Philippines as a structure, since it is not the framework that guides the development of informal settlements. Rather, the agents control the fundamental mechanism that shapes localities, even to the extent of violating the stipulations in the slum upgrading framework. Besides, the dealings, conflicts, and compromises that characterize slum upgrading often take place between agents, and not between structures. The general tone of this presentation has been relatively generalizing, more of a sketching of collective contexts rather than a journey into local specifics that characterizes the manuscript on which this chapter is based.

Nevertheless, it is within these economic, social, and physical dimensions that we must seek to understand the processes by which individuals and groups are bound together in an ongoing process of personal and social actualization. In all, the presentation has demonstrated that, contrary to the idea of the "culture of poverty," which perceives the urban poor as merely passive recipients of urban problems, they are rational, innovative, and nearly always more perceptive than they are often given credit for. As concerned agents of change, the urban poor improvise in order to adapt to a given condition. This culture of improvisation is shown in how they utilize available space, in how they acquire materials for their houses, in the names they call their localities, and in the kind of life that they live.

STATUS ON DHARAVI

Why does the world constantly turn its media, literary, and cinematic attention, not to the cultural legacies of Agra and Thanjavur, but to Dharavi, Asia's so-called "biggest slum"? The answer: we detect some greatness in Dharavi's against-all-odds achievements. Many are drawing back the curtain of slum stereotypes that have prevented insight into the genius in Mumbai's centre of bootstrap poverty reduction. India's cities will double in population over the next 30 years. In ten years, some 20 million new migrants, largely poor, will join the 62 million slum dwellers recognized today.

The nation's prosperity, and perhaps even its stability, hinges on a strategy for urban growth that enables shack-dwelling new arrivals to steadily build a secure, productive, and legal place in the mainstream of urban India. Dharavi shows a way. Its brilliance can be reverse engineered, made systematic, and scaled across the slum-building stand-off that is urban India. So make an audacious proposal: that Dharavi not only be preserved and steadily upgraded, but be designated a United Nations World Heritage Site to protect it from expedient development schemes that would deny India the exemplar of one of its native forms of urbanism.

The United Nations applies four main criteria when selecting districts in cities like Havana, Liverpool, Quito, and Prague for World Heritage Site protection. Dharavi scores high on all accounts. Dharavi exhibits an important interchange of human values on architecture, town-planning and landscape design. In Dharavi, hundredfold chains of migration have mixed very diverse Indian village traditions and trial-and-error approaches to "town planning" to create a global manufacturing and trading city in a matter of decades. Dharavi is a living "interchange of human values" fixed in space and given robust economic logic.

Formal sector urban development today is capital-intensive, and therefore inaccessible to the majority. But unconstrained by large fixed capital investments and maintenance costs, Dharavi's resident-builders practice a flexible, resilient, just-in-time approach to city building that still works at the scale of more than half a million. Dharavi's approach offers two special advantages. First, it is accessible to migrants with limited cash-flow and credit, who incrementally build and upgrade as they generate savings over a period of years.

Second, building design and arrangements can be adapted quickly and efficiently to respond to economic, social, and environmental pressures, offering resilience for those living at the margins. Dharavi demonstrates an economically robust form of city building that allows the poorest to develop complex industrial economies, supporting remittance lifelines across village India from their positive balance of trade.

Dharavi is an outstanding example of a traditional human settlement, bearing unique testimony to a cultural tradition. Like the traditional *mahalles* of western Asia and the *kampungs* of Southeast Asia, Dharavi represents India's tradition of adapting village form, life, and culture into a settlement solution for large cities. These traditional forms of urban settlement smoothen the transition from agricultural to urban society, providing governable and, when necessary, self-reliant social and political units in fast-growing cities.

There are many more modern, yet failed alternatives to organizing large migrant populations, among them the high-rise public housing ghettos in America's inner cities and on France's urban peripheries. With no economic logic of their own (other than constant subsidy), these approaches create centres of instability. Dharavi is an outstanding example of a type of building, architectural ensemble, or landscape that illustrates a significant stage in human history. Just as old Manchester evolved unique building types and ensembles to support the Industrial Revolution, Dharavi evolves urban designs at the front-line of the migratory urban revolution. Every building, shop, and space responds to the lean economics of the migrant city builder.

Otherwise separated buildings and building uses are clustered to support a variety of functions in the same space. There are residential-retail crèche buildings, retail-warehouse-movie theatre buildings, or industrial-residential-warehouse buildings. Dharavi has invented its own form of 24/7, resulting in an extremely high utilization rate of property. Dharavi's residents and businesses also have extremely low costs for transportation. Most of Dharavi's workforce lives there. The alternative is commuting from distant low-cost settlements. Similarly, many Dharavi industries have minimal logistics complexity or cost because manufacturers are located next door to suppliers and retailers.

With low transportation costs, efficient utilization of property, reduced logistics, and clustered entrepreneurial communities, the resident-worker-entrepreneurs of Dharavi gain stable competitive advantage. They can support and educate their families on low wages and long hours, and meanwhile gain access to global finance, goods, and labour markets. Dharavi is directly and tangibly associated with events or living traditions, ideas, or beliefs of outstanding universal significance. The issue of Dharavi's preservation is not about an aged slum. It's about a strategic choice facing India and other rapidly urbanizing countries.

Will New India honour the ingenuity of its urban traditions, and evolve these into even better home-grown solutions? Or will India build its future with less robust solutions imported from other places? The wrong choice can lead to costly folly. The recent sub prime crisis, like the Asian financial crisis before it (1997-1998), is about more than a failure of the banking industry. Both crises were rooted in uncritical acceptance of capital-intensive, industrial-scale models of urban development based on deeply flawed economics during periods of rapid urban growth. Both the Asian Tigers and the US turned away from tested, resilient forms of native urbanism and towards expedient, "modern" ways to become the "next Shanghai" or "next Silicon Valley."

But Dharavi reminds us that effective urbanism provides far more than an expedient fix: it creates places that can be affordably adapted and improved upon to renew competitive advantages in the face of constant change, even for the poorest of households in the hardest of times. Dharavi offers too much guidance to a world of growing cities to face "renewal" through demolition. That is why it captivates the million-fold migrants of India and, with them, the attention of the world. Just as cities like Barcelona, Lisbon, and Rio de Janeiro preserved their erstwhile slum districts as they legalised and invested in them, Dharavi should be proudly claimed and upgraded in partnership with its existing residents. It is a unique and salient creation of living Indian heritage.

8

Women's lives in Sri Lanka

Gender and Culture

The lives of the women, mothers and widows who remain displaced still are arduous, declares Tamil Centre for Human Rights, (TCHR), a human rights watchdog group of the Tamils of Sri Lanka. The Tamil Centre for Human Rights which is based in Paris, France, in a statement issued on the occasion of the International Women's day TCHR further adds: "Displacement impacts on women most significantly through increased workloads, increased psychological and physical health problems. Access to food, safe water and sanitation, essential to maintain health and life, continues to be difficult for many of the displaced women and their families. Thousands still cannot return to their homes, obstructed by the Sri Lankan army. Many of these families have been displaced fifteen or more times."

The full text of the statement issued by *Tamil Centre for Human Rights* is given below:

Today, all over the world, women speak out, wanting to give shape to a world free from gender based poverty, violence and inequality. The *UN Convention on the Elimination of Discrimination Against Women* (CEDAW) has been in existence for nearly a quarter of a century, and now its optional protocol provides a mechanism for individual complaints - but discrimination against women persists. According to UN statistics, women perform two thirds of the world's work;

produce, process and market three fifths of the world's food, but receive only one-tenth of the world's income and own less than one-hundredth of the world's prosperity. In many countries the low value attached to girls results in discrimination and exclusion. Illegal international trafficking of women and girls tricks and coerces thousands into slavery, forcing them to work as prostitutes.

Violence against women is prevalent in many societies and countries. Many incidents are unreported by the victims due to the trauma, shame and fear of stigma. However, violence against women is no longer invisible, due to the determined work of many organizations over the years. The resolution on Women, Peace and Security adopted unanimously by the UN Security Council on October 31, 2000 was a historic victory for women.

As early as 1914, women's NGOs demanded that the rape of women by soldiers in wartime be considered a crime in all countries. Now, under the Rome Statute of the International Criminal Court, systematic rape in wartime has finally been recognized as a crime against humanity. In the island of Sri Lanka rape has been used systematically as a weapon of war by Sri Lankan armed forces. In fact TCHR documented many such cases, prior to the Ceasefire Agreement of February 2002. TCHR established that; a Tamil woman was raped every 16 days; a Tamil woman was gang-raped and murdered every two months; a girl-child was raped every three months and a woman was brutally murdered every six months because she resisted the advances of a Sri Lankan soldier. These horrific statistics are based on documented cases. Real figures are believed to be considerably higher.

Now, since the Ceasefire Agreement has been in place, the situation for Tamil women is improved, however the situation is far from satisfactory. In October last year a 42-year-old women living in Vavuniya went to graze her cattle and never returned home. Her body was found near the local Sri Lanka army camp. The post-mortem revealed that she had been raped and strangled to death. Sri Lanka navy personnel in Nedunthivu (Delft), Jaffna, attempted to rape a mother of four children in December 2002, while she was praying in church. Two Sri Lanka army soldiers forcibly broke into a woman's home in Ganesapuram, Vavuniya, and attempted to rape her in January 2003.

The Tamil women in the North East, who underwent so many hardships and faced so many obstacles earlier, are relieved to be under the present local legal system. This local system prevents abusive power over women through the dowry system and punishes violations against women. The lives of the women, mothers and widows who remain displaced still are arduous. Displacement impacts on women most significantly through increased workloads, increased psychological and physical health problems. Access to food, safe water and sanitation, essential to maintain health and life, continues to be difficult for many of the displaced women and their families.

Thousands still cannot return to their homes, obstructed by the Sri Lankan army. Many of these families have been displaced fifteen or more times. So, in the island that produced the World's first woman Prime Minister and currently has a woman President, it is with sadness that we are compelled to note the ongoing pain and suffering that thousands of Tamil women are experiencing still today. Let us hope that justice will reign and that respect and dignity will triumph. Let us hope for a future in which all the human rights of women and the political aspirations of the Tamil people in their homeland in the North East of the island will be respected and fulfilled. Only then can there be durable peace.

More importantly, the country's economy rests to a very large part on the shoulders of women. The Sri Lankan economy's main foreign exchange earners used to be tea, rubber and coconut cultivation for export. Apart from these commercial crops, paddy (rice) cultivation has been the mainstay of the rural economy. Women's labour plays an important role here, but in most instances is not taken into account. The traditional economic pattern has completely changed during the last 10-15 years. Remittances from Sri Lankans employed in the Middle Eastern countries are now the no.1 net foreign exchange earner and women constitute more than 80% of this work-force. In earning this money, women have to go undergo a great deal of hardship.

Firstly, even to leave Sri Lanka for these jobs, they are exploited by the so-called employment agencies. Sometimes they charge Rs.30-40,000 (£3-4,000) to send a woman abroad for a housemaid's job. But the real trauma only starts after they reach the country and start the job. The women have no fixed hours of work, proper health care facilities etc. They are at the mercy of their employers. This situation is not only limited to housemaids. Recently a Sri Lankan employee of a garment factory in Saudi Arabia was suspended from work. The other workers, mostly women, walked out in solidarity, though they were not organized in a union. All of them were instantly dismissed.

The Sri Lankan authorities took no action to protect these workers on the pretext that striking was illegal in Saudi Arabia. The actual reason was that the Sri Lankan authorities did not want to offend the feudal rulers and big business in the Saudi kingdom. There have been numerous other instances where women employees have been victimised, beaten, sexually abused and even killed. Most women are afraid to divulge the incidents due to the stigma attached to them.

Even when they are reported, little or nothing is done by the Sri Lankan government but in February this year it had to intervene to bring back about 200 Sri Lankan women from Lebanon. They had were stranded after being dismissed by their employers after just 3-4 months employment. They had not been paid their salaries and a considerable number arrived in wheelchairs, showing the trauma they had undergone at the hands of their employers or agencies.

The tea plantations in Sri Lanka account for two thirds of all plantations and employ a very large number of women but almost all in unskilled or semi-skilled work such as plucking tea-leaves, sweeping and collecting tea dust, etc. Up to mid-1980 women workers were discriminated against, receiving lower wages than men for the same type of work. Although that has been formally remedied, they still work in semi-slave conditions comprising illiteracy, malnutrition and improper sanitation. Almost all plantation workers are organized in trade unions but the number of women holding positions in them is negligible and they have not taken up specific issues affecting women workers.

The garment industry, which has spread throughout the country during the last 10 years, is another sector where a large number of women are employed - constituting about 80% of the work-force and occupying the lowest grades. The basic salary of a machine operator is between Rs.2,500 and Rs.3,500 - very low by comparison with other comparable vocations and with the magnitude of the income and profit of these enterprises, This industry is hugely invested in by foreign businesses simply because of the greater possibilities of exploiting an educated work-force. Although Sri Lanka has a relatively strong trade union tradition, the garment sector does not allow trade union rights.

These workers have still not been organized and the left movement has not been able to fill this vacuum. There are several 'Free Trade Zones' (or Export Promotion Zones) in the country where foreign investment has concentrated, originally mainly in the garment industry but now also in others like diamond cutting, footwear and rubber-based industries. The FTZs, which allow investors huge tax benefits and other concessions, employ women to a very large extent. The Korean and Japanese firms - the main foreign investors - only want to collect a big profit in a short period. Thereafter they vanish, abandoning the factory and workers without paying their salaries and other statutory payments due to them.

At present there is an agitation by a group of workers in this situation - the majority of them are women in a Korean-owned establishment called Kabool Magnetic. The government is not taking any action over the dispute. In these FTZ factories, working women's rights are zero - not only trade union rights but basic human rights. One example is that women workers wanting to go to the toilet have to wait to get a card and mark the time on it. They call it the 'piss card' and many women get health problems because of the system. There is a continuous agitation taking place against these inhuman practices.

The stereotype woman still promoted by some in Sri Lanka is the house-wife and mother who cares for the husband and children by cooking, washing and house-keeping. But the changed situation, after the economy was opened up to 'free' market forces in the late '70s, has compelled every woman to seek employment just to bear house-hold expenses. The majority of women have become economically less dependent and that has raised their position *vis-à-vis* men in society. On the other hand, women are being exploited extensively as their jobs are at lower grades and mostly of an unskilled or semi-skilled nature. The professions of teaching and nursing are also more than 70% female as these jobs are traditionally considered as appropriate for women. However, here also a comparatively low percentage of women occupy higher positions.

The Sri Lankan constitution of 1978 formally guarantees equal legal rights for women. Nevertheless some traditional laws such as thesawalamai (of Northern Hindus) and Muslim law still discriminate against women as do immigration laws. If a Sri Lankan woman decides to marry a foreigner, she will not be able to get him citizenship rights whereas a Sri Lankan man will get citizenship rights for a foreign wife automatically, 'ipso facto'.

The darkest side of women's lives is the alarming increase in violence against them reported in the last few years - rape, other forms of sexual abuse and even murder. A particular scandal is that young working girls in the free trade zones have become prey for the perpetrators of sexual crimes including many soldiers of the Sri Lankan army. Though there is a new awareness and emphasis on women's rights, violence against women has not abated. Domestic violence is traditionally accepted as a part of married life.

There are now a considerable number of households where the only bread-winners are women and many of them are single parents. This has increased as a result of the war in the north and the east of the country where a Tamil minority is fighting for the right to self-determination and also of the youth rebellion in the south in the late eighties. There is no proper social security network for these women, apart from some ad hoc measures. Though women's role in the economy and society has become more and more important, her position is still vulnerable. There is no clear and general identification and recognition of women's rights as human rights.

The previous UNP government published a women's charter embodying various women's rights recognized internationally. The present PA government, led by two women, pledged at the elections in 1994 to legalize that charter. However, no action has been taken in that regard, despite there being a Women's Affairs Ministry led by a woman. Unfortunately, the traditional left movement and trade unions also have not taken up women's issues seriously and effectively. They have had the concept that women's rights and problems are only a part of the social issues in general, many saying that the social transformation of society will automatically resolve them.

However, women's issues have surfaced prominently now and Non Governmental Organizations have become the main bodies active in this arena. They have played a useful role but they have not been able to address the real issues of the exploitation perpetrated by capitalism. Also, NGOs never put the class issues forward. There is an urgent need for the left movement to take up women's issues as a priority matter and fight for equality, for an end to discrimination, exploitation and the oppression of women.

URBAN SLUMS

The project is designed to assist Governments to lead and coordinate technical cooperation and seed capital initiatives to develop bankable projects that promote affordable housing for low- income households. SUF is being piloted in four countries in Asia and Africa with Sri Lanka being one of these four countries. Initiating the second SUF project in Sri Lanka, the project finance advisor for SUF Ms. Angela Mwai expressed her view by saying, "In developing countries urban slums have been a developing problem.

If we think about the urban slums around the world, they are mainly located in central parts of the major cities. Therefore, for the urban development upgrading urban slums becomes crucial. The economic factor becomes a barrier in upgrading slums around the world. However, LFSUS was established in order to facilitate the financial issue with the participation of public and private stakeholders". The central objective of SUF is to assist developing countries to attract domestic capital for their slum upgrading and related infrastructure activities.

Dr. P. Ramanujam, Secretary of Ministry of Urban Development and Sacred Area Development, expressed his gratitude to HNB for the willingness to grant loans to this project jointly with UN-HABITAT, LFSUS and Sri Lanka Women's Development Services Cooperative Society (WOMEN'S BANK) and thanked Chandula P. Abeywickrema, Deputy General Manager of HNB and Chairman of LFSUS who has been the "Leading Light" in the HNB Banking Sector for inaugurating this venture to serve the community of our country. The main purpose of this project is to help the people especially in urban rural areas to open a new perspective in their lives, by way of providing opportunities to develop their business, jobs and also to assist in obtaining housing loans etc. We need institutes like these in Sri Lanka which can contribute to and stimulate its national growth in the country.

INFRASTRUCTURE

The Kuruniyawatta project is located in the outskirts of the Shell-Gas Road off Kolonnawa main junction within Kolonnawa MC. The total population of the entire settlement is 235 and their livelihood options comprise working as

Municipal Council labourers, three-wheeler drivers, and other small scale, low-income business men. It is a multi ethnic community inclusive of Sinhalese, Tamils, Muslims, Malays and other ethnic minorities. The proposed development of the Kuruniyawatta settlement will take place on site as the same land will be utilized for the development process. Since most of the infrastructure is available within the settlement, the project will upgrade the existing houses within the limited area space.

Sri Lanka, The Pearl Of the Indian Ocean, has made steady progress since the opening of its economy in 1977. But the poor have seen few of the benefits. Policies to alleviate poverty and development efforts by the government and international non-governmental organizations have been hampered by three decades on civil war. More than four million people are estimated to live below the poverty line with about half a million of them residing in slums and shanties.

There is now cause for optimism if, as expected, the government's push into eastern and northern areas occupied by the *Liberation Tigers of Tamil Elam* brings an end to the conflict. Development was set back by the Indian Ocean tsunami in 2004 which left 100,000 homeless. The country is still recovering as reconstruction continues in the badly hit Eastern Province. Rehabilitation is still needed in the Northern Province.

Sri Lanka is highly rural; only one-in-five people lives in towns and cities. Rural dwellers lack access to water, sanitation, electricity, communication, roads and other infrastructure and services. The rural poor often live in makeshift shacks constructed of mud and discarded materials that offer scant protection from the weather and wildlife. Children living in these unsafe structures " which are damp, moldy and need constant maintenance are often sick.

Shelter conditions for urban dwellers are no better. The influx of rural workers seeking jobs in the capital city of Colombo, has contributed to the growth of slums. The United

Nations cites a shortage of affordable low-cost housing for low-income people as a major reason for the growth of such informal settlements. According to UN-HABITAT, more than half of the 2.3 million people living in Colombo live in slum conditions. Overcrowding is common. A five-member family in such areas has to make do with an average of less than 32 sq. m. (350 sq. ft.) of space. Typically, slum residents do not have legal rights to the land they occupy.

The government has two major initiatives to address substandard housing: the Million Houses Programme and Urban Basic Services Programme. These programmes draw on community-based organizations to leverage local participation in shelter and infrastructure improvements. The government has also granted tenure to slum residents and increased investment in infrastructure. Still, more needs to be done. By 2010, Sri Lanka is expected to face a shortage of some 650,000 homes, excluding those built for families affected by the tsunami. By then, about half of the population is expected to be living in urban slums.

Habitat for Humanity began operating in Sri Lanka in 1994, through affiliates. The model later evolved into a series of Habitat Resource Centers that support satellite centers and individual projects in four regions. Today, HFH Sri Lanka is probably the country's largest home builder after the government. The former affiliate, now satellite center, in Anuradhapura pioneered Habitat's housing microfinance scheme, Save & Build, in 2000. This sees groups of about 12 families saving toward the cost of one house. When that amount is reached, Habitat matches their efforts with a loan to build two more houses, thus allowing three houses to be built. The cycle repeats until each group member has a house. Loan repayments are recycled into a fund to help other savings groups.

HFH Sri Lanka's builds two-room core house covers about 24 sq. m. Under the Building in Stages model, once the initial mortgage is repaid, a second loan is taken out to finance a second section " either a third room or a verandah is added, increasing the size to 32 sq. m. To reduce construction costs, savings group members make bricks as well as gather raw materials. Habitat houses are kept affordable through the help of volunteer labor. Since the tsunami, HFH Sri Lanka has hosted more than 1,000 volunteers. More than 50 teams worked on post-tsunami reconstruction sites and more than 30 Global Village teams have built on regular sites.

Specialist construction teams, and 35 corporate teams sent by HFH Great Britain in partnership with UK-based community challenge were among those to work on post-tsunami projects. Habitat also works with partners such as non-governmental organizations World Concern, World Vision, Tearfund and Christian Aid, as well as the United States Agency for International Development, and church groups.

9

Slums of India and Gender

Slums...the picture that conjures up in our minds is that of a dirty, unhygienic group of make shift shanties with long lines of people waiting at the Municipal water pump, bawling babies literally left on street corners to fend for themselves and endless cries of help. When did India slide into this chaos? According to a recently conducted survey, 22% of Indian urban population lives in slums as against 32% for the whole world population; most, if not all of these people earn under the urban poverty line. Data from a study by National Institute of Urban Affairs (NIUA) reported that among the poorest cities were Calcutta (89% below the poverty line), Bangalore (73%) and Indore (68%).

More disturbingly, there was a gender divide in the distribution of urban poor in the slums: NIUA reported that 68% of this group consisted of women. Also notable is the fact that 6 million of this population is in the age group 0-6. If we consider a specific case of the glittering metropolis of Mumbai, it appears that 55% of the total population of 11 million is slum dwellers occupying about 12.85% of the city's total land area. There has been an increase of 4% in the number of households living in one-room tenements in the span of a decade, 1981 to 1991 (Government of Maharashtra, 1995).

Also, 8.5 million of the city's population lives in sub-standard or unsafe housing conditions under the continuous threat of displacement. Are Slums a Problem? From a mainstream view, it can be said that slums "spoil" the look of the city. Because slums breed poverty and high unemployment, there is a high crime rate stemming from these neighborhoods. Since these are illegal settlements on encroached public land, they do not pay the basic or civic utilities taxes expected from any legal settlements in a city.

However to be fair, we should consider the prevalent conditions in these urban slums from another viewpoint- slums have inhuman and dangerous living conditions with a total lack of security and a fear of demolition at any point. They do not have basic civic services like waste collection and disposal, clean drinking water, properly maintained drainage system, electricity or paved roads. Take the issue of equitable distribution of municipal water: even in cities claiming 100 percent coverage, the per capita availability varies 10 times between poor/slum and rich locations. For instance, in Ahmedabad, 25% of the population consumed 90% of the water while the rest 75% had to do with only 10%.

Sanitary conditions are literally non-existent in slums: infant mortality rates are higher by 1.8 times in slums as compared to non-slum areas. It has been reported that nearly 50% of urban child mortality is the result of poor sanitation and lack of access to clean drinking water in the urban slums. Slum dwellers constantly live with the fear of losing their home (sometimes they invest thousands to build these) and their possessions to demolishers. Many settlements have been demolished again and again, even though they were built before 1995, which according to the government are legal houses.

In spite of many of these people having proper documentation (ration cards, Vote ID cards) to prove their domicile legally, there has been no respite. In this whole rigmarole of demolitions and re-settlements, huge amounts of money pass hands as bribe to the police, goons and corporations. Also, these demolitions are not preceded by proper notices; India, as a signatory to UN Human Rights treaty is bound to follow certain procedure before any evictions. Hear it first hand from one of these slum dwellers: "I used to live in Tatanagar in Govandi. For the past seven or eight years, not have any problem with water, as 14 of us shared a tap. Before that, we had to go quite a distance. The municipality had provided five taps, but there was no road beside the tracks to reach them.

So we had to walk between the tracks for 10–15 minutes. There used to be lots of fights for filling water. We had to queue for as long as an hour and we had to leave our children behind. Once, my small daughter walked out of the house and sat on the railway track. There used to be many people who came to fill the water and they came from far. For toilets, we had to use the railway tracks. There were public toilets, but they were some distance away - about half an hour walk. They used to be so dirty that we did not feel like using them.

And there were such long queues! Instead of using those filthy toilets, we used to go on the tracks after ten at night or early in the morning at four or five o'clock." What leads to this booming increase in slum settlements in a city: think rapid and uncontrolled Urbanisation which is intimately connected with migration from suburban and rural areas, think the unavailability of basic minimum wages and basic perks (like affordable housing schemes) for these people. What has the Government done to tackle this? So, what is the solution to this? Evictions and demolitions have been seen by the state as one of the major solutions to the "problems" of slums.

The rights of slum dweller to shelter, basic amenities, etc. have also been marginally and occasionally addressed. There has been no consistent or unified Government policy through the 50's till the 90's except for a policy of brute force demolition. For example, section 354A was introduced to the Bombay Municipal Corporation (BMC) Act in 1954 that empowered the Municipal Corporation of Mumbai to clear slums in a totalitarian fashion.

In 1956, the then central Government approved a Slum Clearance Plan. Bombay was one of the six pilot cities covered under this scheme which would lead to blatant use of force to clear these tenements. According to the Maharashtra Vacant

Lands (Prohibition of Unauthorized Structures and Summary Eviction) Act, 1975 all land encroached by squatters can be considered vacant, and all slums covered by the Act can be removed. What's more...the "squatters" have to pay 'compensation' for unauthorized occupation of land. However, the realization dawned slowly that demolition and re-settlement is not the answer.

Resettlement in most cases proceeded erratically and was dependent on the whims and fancies of local municipal officials and the affected poor were completely excluded from any decision-making. This led to the Slum Improvement Programme in the 70's to improve the basic amenities like drainage, drinking water, roads, toilets etc. However, the 80's again saw another spate of demolitions in Mumbai; on a positive note, the Supreme court ruled that eviction of the petitioners (slum dwellers) will lead to deprivation of their livelihood and consequently to the deprivation of their life and violates Article 21.

The story continues with the efforts of the Government and policy makers at the top; however, no one really asks the people who have been affected on what their position is. The Slum Upgrading Programme (SUP) funded by the World Bank in 1985 covered only 22,000 households and was terminated in 1994. The Slum Redevelopment Scheme (1991) provided some new incentives for private developers and builders to redevelop slums– such as the ability to transfer development rights to other areas of the city.

The theory was that by selling the extra space in the open market, tenements for slum dwellers would be cross-subsidized and made affordable to them. However, this was a big non-starter due to the existing skepticism of the slum dwellers for developer/builders, given their history of forcible evictions in the past; on the other hand, the builders themselves did not think this to be a good business opportunity nor did they anticipate a good return on their investment. 1995 saw the Slum Rehabilitation Scheme, an election promise by the Shiv Sena that would provide free tenements to 4 million slum dwellers.

However, this also bit dust as only about 19,000 tenements were completed finally. The Shivshahi Punarvasan Prakalp Ltd that was constituted in 1998 to provide re-settlement actually turned to be a scheme that enriched Mumbai's powerful construction lobby by robbing both public assets and the urban poor (S.S. Tinaikar Committee, 2001). In 2001, the Government and NGOs formulated the slum resettlement plan for 60,000 people.

The Draft National Slum Policy of 2001 initiated a newer level of understanding of the issue of urban slums- that slums are an integral part of urban areas and contribute significantly to their economy both through their labor market contributions and informal production activities. Rather than looking at slums as "problem areas" which need "corrective action", local bodies should recognize the contribution made by slums and make sufficient provision for them to have access to affordable land, housing sites and services.

It was carried out with popular participation and partnerships with NGOs that had been involved in the recent Mumbai Urban Transport Project. The resettled families had a mixed response. On the one hand they were happy to have secure tenure and access to basic services but on the other hand the resettlement location offered fewer employment opportunities and led to increased travel costs for quite a few. On the whole, this policy broadens the definition of slums to include all under-serviced areas. It does not advocate slum clearance policies except under strict resettlement & rehabilitation guidelines which are defined in respect of slums located on untenable sites.

The different issues that should be kept in mind when dealing with in situ resettlement and rehabilitation plans of urban slums include: affordable housing, security of tenure, innovative and cost-effective designs, assurance of basic amenities, and most of all community participation. All urban informal settlements should have access to certain basic minimum services irrespective of land tenure or occupancy status.

The major areas that still need to be addressed to have a clear policy on urban slums include: town planning, land management, poverty alleviation, basic service delivery and capacity building. "It's a momentous victory for the indefatigable spirit of the *Bhopalis*. This campaign showed that the world is watching and the governments cannot flee from taking responsibility of its own citizens," - Kirankumar Vissa, Director, Association for India's Development.

A long fought well deserved victory. The never-say-die spirit of the people affected by the Bhopal Gas disaster has finally paid off. 21 years after the world's worst industrial disaster at a Union Carbide pesticide factory in Bhopal, *Bhopalis* finally made Government of India accept their just demands for justice and a life of dignity. The survivors and other residents have been denied even basic amenities like access to clean drinking water.

Neither Dow Chemical (which fully acquired Union Carbide and its liabilities) nor Government of India has addressed the situation in Bhopal. 51 *Bhopalis* affected by the disaster along with three activists from ICJB (International Campaign for Justice in Bhopal), marched 800 km on foot to Delhi to achieve their long awaited redressal. The month-long march started on February 20, 2006 and was followed by an indefinite hunger strike by *padayatris* at Delhi; *Bhopalis* set forth six demands to the Government of India:

1. Set up a national commission to improve health and economic conditions of the gas affected
2. Provide safe drinking water
3. Prosecute Union Carbide and Warren Anderson
4. Make Dow clean up the factory and pay for it
5. Stop Government purchase of Dow products and halt any expansion of Dow's business in India till it accepts the pending liabilities in Bhopal.
6. Commemorate the disaster with full involvement of the survivors and make the disaster a part of school curriculum

In support of the Bhopal survivors, concerned Americans and Indian Diaspora from 17 cities across the US (Washington DC, New York, Boston, Austin, Houston, Philadelphia, Seattle, San Francisco, San Diego, Atlanta, Tempe, Minneapolis, Cincinnati, Baltimore, Princeton, Ann Arbor and Chicago) initiated demonstrations and vigils. Bhopal Support groups in the United States called and emailed the Indian Embassy and Consulates in the US, since February 20th, urging the Indian government to address the issues raised by the *Bhopalis*.

Over 400 international supporters pledged to fast for at least a day in solidarity with the Bhopal hunger strikers and bombarded the Prime Ministers office in Delhi with over 3000 faxes. On the seventh day of their indefinite hunger strike, the Bhopal survivors called off their protests as the Prime Minister conceded to four of the six long-standing demands on April 17, 2006.

The Prime Minister did not agree to prosecute the multinational corporation and its CEO and also refused to halt the expansion of Dow until it accepts its liabilities. In the latest development, JDA, under the supervision of the Hon'ble High Court of Rajasthan, has offered alternative sites for relocating the Bandhyali School. *Digantar* has accepted one such relocation schemes, but the details are yet to be finalized.

Universalizing primary education may be a major goal of the Government policy makers. But the Jaipur Development Authority (JDA) curiously seems unaware of this. It has issued a notice to demolish a school providing free education to poor and deprived kids for the past 12 years. The school is located in Bandhyali, a village 20 kms from Jaipur, where land prices have tripled in the past one year. The primary school, established in 1992, with financial support from the Ministry of Human Resource Development, has been providing education to over 300 children, mostly girls from very poor and backward families (in Kho Nagoriyan and Bhavgarh Bandhya villages) since 1993.

All of the children are from educationally and socio-economically disadvantaged sections of society such as *Malis*,

Muslims and Gujjars. *Digantar,* the voluntary organisation that runs the Bandhyali and other neighboring schools, is known nationally for its innovative curriculum and pedagogy and is visited annually by a large number of educationists, teachers and voluntary organizations. *Digantar* has been working since 1978 in the field of education and its areas of work include framing of curriculum, alternative pedagogy for elementary education and teachers' development. It has contributed to several innovative national endeavors including *Lok Jumbish* in Rajasthan, the alternative schools of the Rajiv Gandhi Siksha Mission in Madhya Pradesh, and textbook development of NCERT.

However, in a blatant violation of the Fundamental Right to "free and compulsory education" granted to every child in the age group of 6-14 years under Article 21A, the JDA issued a notice to *Digantar* in December asking them to vacate the land. It seems that JDA has unilaterally reserved this land for allotment to "Mahima Shiksha Samiti" for setting up a private university. With the JDA ordering the school to be demolished, students are deeply concerned about their future. "I want to become a doctor but if this school shuts down I don't know where I will study. My parents will not send me to any other school as they trust only this one. If it closes I will remain uneducated," said a student.

Another student said, "I am scared because my parents will not send me to any other school. My elder brothers and sisters have all studied here. All other schools are very far." As Rohit Dhankar, the Director of *Digantar,* points out, "It is not a question of one small school closing down. It is a question of children in this country receiving their fundamental rights to education. If this school shuts down, these children will have to stay at home. They have nowhere else to go." For Bandhyali villagers and *Digantar,* the land per se is not important. What is critically important is that the school continues, so that children have access to meaningful education. For JDA, however, this land seems important only as a commercial resource.

In the wake of tremendous public mobilization against this notice, *Digantar,* with the help of the community and various NGOs and concerned citizens moved the Hon'ble High Court of Rajasthan and got a stay order directing the JDA to first consider its long- pending application for allotment of land. Your help is needed to ensure that Bandhyali School is not sacrificed to a unilateral decision of the JDA to promote privatization of education at the cost of free primary education for minority children. Let's take the example of a village with around 200 houses. 150 of them don't have electricity, though the village is officially "electrified".

You investigate, and find out from the villagers that the only way to obtain an electricity connection would be to pay a fairly large bribe, say some 1500 rupees. This may not seem too exorbitant, but we're talking about very poor villagers, who spend about 40 rupees per month on kerosene for their lanterns. Many of them want electricity so that they can have a couple of light bulbs at home, their kids can stay back and study in the evenings, and perhaps they can afford a fan to use in the summer months. Seems very basic, but this small change means a lot to them.

And they cannot afford to pay the bribe, and remain powerless (pardon the pun). The situation was thrown open to us, and we were asked for possible solutions. Here are some that were voiced.

1. Try to unite the poor villagers, and force the local authorities to provide the villagers these basic services by taking legal action against them. Problems with this scenario: This would certainly be a long and difficult struggle. If you as an outsider were doing this, you will have to remain in this village for a long time (probably years) to see this fight through. Secondly, the villagers might have to undergo a lot of other hardships (repercussions) if they start these demands. Thirdly, it is difficult to keep a group already with difficulties to stay united. Legal disputes take a long time for resolution in court (years sometimes), and can be very expensive. Who

will bear the expense for that many years? Who will ensure the implementation of the court verdict?

2. We know that such corruption exists. But there is some validity of strength in numbers. So, couldn't the villagers unite, and then say that though they can't pay the huge bribe, they will together pool a smaller (but still large, because of scale up) amount each, and give this in bulk. Sort of like a Costco or Sam's club bulk rate pricing, a discounted rate of corruption (yes, a couple of us came up with this idea!) Problems with this scenario: Come on, if an ethical battle is being fought, you have to take a correct stand. This would absolutely condone corruption. Additionally, it may or may not work, but will make any future in the progress next to impossible.
3. As an NGO, promote alternate energy sources, such as solar or biogas, which can be used in place of electricity. Problems with this scenario: This one can be viable, but only in certain cases. The costs of solar lightning etc are much higher than conventional electricity sources, and require a lot of funding. It is cheaper for say, solar cookers, but solar lighting is another proposition all together. With biogas etc, it's not enough to have cattle, but there should be a certain number of cattle, as well as sufficient quantities of water to spare. Again, cost factors are fairly high (to build a distribution system etc). However, some groups, like the Barefoot college have managed to solve some problems with this approach. Still, it is difficult for small groups to do this in a large number of villages. Implementation requires a huge grassroots base, which most groups don't have.
4. Look for sincere officials to help combat these problems. After all, all government officials can't be bad. Problems with this scenario: It is absolutely true that there are good government and administrative officials, who are not corrupt and work sincerely. However, they are not the rule, and a large section of the officials are not in this category. Often, the good ones are themselves powerless given their surroundings (if say there is a good middle

level official, but the immediate superior is corrupt, the good official is unable to act. Sometimes, a junior official who is corrupt might be politically or locally very powerful, and the senior official can't go against him/her). But it certainly is a good idea to find these officials, and take their help whenever possible. However, in, say the situation above, this alone will not provide a solution.

5. Gather some villagers, surround (in this case) the linesman and ask him why he accepts bribes (say at a *panchayat* meeting). Try to publicly question him, and hope that yields results. Problems with this scenario: Usually, the lowest official will claim that he's being paid too little. Then the villagers will clamor that this is not true, and reveal his (usually rather adequate) salary. He'll backtrack, and then say that his share of the bribe in only 50 rupees, the rest go to superiors. So he might magnanimously forfeit his share. But this gets more and more difficult as you go up the ladder (to say a senior engineer, whose cut is actually heftier). Still, there are merits in this suggestion as well.
6. How about negotiating a settlement with the officials, with a request that they at least consider requests from the poorest applicants without demanding bribes. The list would be provided to the officials by an impartial external group (say the NGO), with the guarantee that each person in the list is too poor to possibly pay the bribe. This person could then be awarded a connection. The carrot to the government officials in this case would be a guarantee not to go to the press, or press charges. Problems with this scenario: Even if the officials agree to this (due to your constant pressure), they might take a very long time to execute this/clear the files. Additionally, would it not be unfair to the others, who, though they can possibly afford the bribe, should by right not have to pay it. Where do you draw the line? Here you are not really condoning corruption, but you are drawing some line to start your fight. However, it is a possibly viable stance.

India's slum population doubles since the 1980s

The number of urban slum-dwellers rose from 27.9 million in 1981 to 46.2 million in 1991 and 61.8 million in 2001, according to estimates by the Town and Country Planning Organisation The number of people living in slums in India, Asia's fourth largest economy and the world's second fastest growing one, has more than doubled in the past two decades, according to official figures.

About a quarter of the country's billion-plus population now live in towns and cities. The number of urban slum-dwellers rose from 27.9 million in 1981 to 46.2 million in 1991 and 61.8 million in 2001 - the latest census data available - according to estimates by Town and Country Planning Organisation, Junior Minister for Housing and Urban Poverty Alleviation, Kumari Selja, told the Rajya Sabha or Upper House of Parliament, on May 17, 2007.

The country's financial capital, Mumbai, houses the largest number of urban slums - some 6.5 million people live in them. The city is also home to Asia's largest slum, Dharavi. New Delhi follows, with 1.8 million people living in squalor, bereft of even the basic necessities of sanitation and clean drinking water. Kolkata, with 1.49 lakh slum inhabitants, is a close third. Although the Indian economy has grown at an average of 8.6% in the last four years, analysts say the growth has not touched millions of India's poor. The government has launched several schemes to provide housing and civic amenities to slum-dwellers in cities, like the Jawaharlal Nehru National Urban Renewal Mission (JNNURM), said Selja.

She added: "The basic services in the urban poor programme address housing and civic amenities in 63 Mission cities." Non-mission Cities are addressed through the Integrated Housing and Slum Development Programme, Selja added. But civil rights groups say the government has not done enough. "Slums are here to stay," says Maju Varghese of YUVA Urban, a social organisation working with the urban poor. "What has happened is the total failure of the government to provide affordable housing to the urban poor. The government has completely ignored this problem."

HEALTHCARE IN URBAN SLUMS IN INDIA

The growth of cities has always been accompanied by the growth of slums. The industrial revolution in Western Europe led to the migration of people to slums in cities, which created new conditions of ill health due to overcrowding, poor housing and unsanitary environment, coupled with poverty. While public health crises were not unknown in earlier times, the institutions of family and church were primarily responsible for care and relief.

Urbanisation broke down those traditional family and community structures and the working class in particular was pushed to the brink of destitution in a crisis such as an epidemic or a natural calamity. It was left to the state (primarily the political and administrative wings) to become the moral 'parent' of the poor. As a part of this role, the health of the urban poor became a subject of enquiry for administrators and planners in the mid-nineteenth century. In India too, when large-scale Urbanisation took place after the First World War, the decades of the 1920s to the 1940s saw an upsurge of research in urban health. These studies were particularly notable for the exploration of the link between poverty, living conditions and ill health.

Ironically, although a substantial proportion of the research on poverty and health emerged from cities in the pre-Independence era, urban health was not at the focus of public health practice in the years after Independence. India was viewed as a largely rural society and, thus, the government's conception of primary healthcare was almost entirely rural oriented. This bias was also not corrected by the voluntary community health movement, which too focused on the problems of providing primary healthcare to the rural poor.

With rapid Urbanisation, as in most developing countries, public health problems in India are increasingly assuming an urban dimension. In the 2001 Census, 27.8% of the population was found to be living in urban areas. Between 1991 and 2001, 14.3 million people were added to the urban population due to migration. In cities with a population over a million, nearly one-fourth (24.1%) of the population was residing in slums.

The recent National Sample Survey also indicates that the proportion of the population living below the poverty line in rural and urban areas equalized in 2004-05. In each, it is estimated that about 22% of the population lives below the poverty line. It has been observed that the decline in poverty has been lower in urban compared with rural areas. Understanding public health needs in urban areas requires a different conceptual framework. Traditionally, it is understood that alleviation of poverty is the most important precursor of improving general health. But in urban areas, the marginal increase in income for the poor, in itself, does not assure better living conditions due to wide disparities, which make decent accommodation, and clean water and air unaffordable.

Moreover, certain necessities, which existed as free goods in rural settings, are commodities in urban areas such as drinking water, cooking fuel, housing space, etc. The poor are typically driven to the margins of the urban space, where living conditions are the most degraded and of little economic value. The relative difference in income and wealth is much starker in urban areas. The higher purchasing power of the rich drives the prices of food and healthcare goods, making them unaffordable to the poor.

The rich also consume more than their fair share of public goods, for example, water, infrastructure, electricity, which are often subsidized by the state. Urban policies and laws look upon migration (particularly of the poor) as the root of the problem. They respond by imposing penalties on the poor in different ways, such as by denying them the right to housing, refusing them a ration card or neglecting to create adequate infrastructure for their use. As a result, slums become the focal points of punitive action, which aggravates the deprivation caused by economic uncertainty faced by those dependent on casual wage labour.

A study found high levels of malnutrition among children below 5 years of age in Mumbai, and the levels of stunting, which is an indicator of long term chronic malnutrition, were almost similar in the sample of the urban poor children as in a sample of tribal children taken from the poverty-stricken Jawhar talukain neighbouring Thane district. This study found that while 17.6% of boys were stunted in urban slums, the figure was 17.8% for the sample of tribal boys in the same age group.

The study concluded that the high levels of stunting in urban areas were not related to food scarcity, but to environmental and social factors such as access to healthcare, clean drinking water, repeated childhood infections, mother's nutrition and her ability to breastfeed. This was related to the uncertain availability of casual wage employment, especially for women. Are view of studies on the situation of reproductive and child health in urban areas noted that there were consistent differences in antenatal care (ANC) coverage between slum and non-slum areas.

While 74% of women in non- slum areas received 3 or more ANC check-ups, only 55% of the women in slums did. This study also found that 27% of infants in slums had a low birth weight compared with 18% of those born in non-slum areas. In addition, there were significant differences in health access among those living in 'recognized' and 'unrecognized' slums. (In Maharashtra, as per the slum rehabilitation policy, slum households can prove his residency before 1 January, 1995 are 'recognized'.) While 78% of women living in the former had an institutional delivery, this figure was only 65% for the latter. While 81% of children in recognized slums received 3 doses of DPT, only 67% of those in unrecognized slums were fully immunized against DPT.

Poverty and other forms of social disadvantage translate into poorer health status and outcomes for the urban poor. There is a need for a comprehensive policy for primary healthcare for urban areas, which takes into account the special concerns of the poor. Such a policy would aim, first, to address the absolute deprivation of basic necessities - food, housing, water supply and sanitation that the urban poor experience.

Second, there is a need to create an adequate and functional network of free services that are non- discriminatory and reach out to all sections of the population.

Finally, an urban health policy would need to address the problem of social inequality in a proactive manner. The urban poor will continue to depend on the market, not merely for healthcare but for all aspects of daily life, including employment and survival needs. The state must recognize its obligation to protect the poor against the vagaries of the market, because of which they are exploited or driven out by the overwhelming influence of the rich.

All cities in India are loud, but nothing matches the 24/7 decibel level of Mumbai, the former Bombay, where the traffic never stops and the horns always honk. Noise, however, is not a problem in Dharavi, the teeming slum of one million souls, where as many as 18,000 people crowd into a single acre (0.4 hectares). By nightfall, deep inside the maze of lanes too narrow even for the putt-putt of auto rickshaws, the slum is as still as a verdant glade. Once you get accustomed to sharing 300 square feet (28 square meters) of floor with 15 humans and an uncounted number of mice, a strange sense of relaxation sets in - ah, at last a moment to think straight.

Dharavi is routinely called "the largest slum in Asia," a dubious attribution sometimes conflated into "the largest slum in the world." This is not true. Mexico City's Neza-Chalco-Itza barrio has four times as many people. In Asia, Karachi's Orangi Township has surpassed Dharavi. Even in Mumbai, where about half of the city's swelling 12 million population lives in what is euphemistically referred to as "informal" housing, other slum pockets rival Dharavi in size and squalor.

Yet Dharavi remains unique among slums. A neighborhood smack in the heart of Mumbai, it retains the emotional and historical pull of a sub continental Harlem - a square-mile (three square kilometers) center of all things, geographically, psychologically, spiritually. Its location has also made it hot real estate in Mumbai, a city that epitomizes India's hopes of becoming an economic rival to China. Indeed, on a planet where half of humanity will soon live in cities, the forces at work in Dharavi serve as a window not only on the future of India's burgeoning cities, but on urban space everywhere.

Ask any longtime resident - some families have been here for three or more generations - how Dharavi came to be, and they'll say, "We built it." This is not far off. Until the late 19th century, this area of Mumbai was mangrove swamp inhabited by Koli fishermen. When the swamp filled in (with coconut leaves, rotten fish, and human waste), the Kolis are deprived of their fishing grounds and they would have to soon shift to bootlegging liquor but room became available for others. The *Kumbhars* came from Gujarat to establish a potters' colony. Tamils arrived from the south and opened tanneries. Thousands traveled from Uttar Pradesh to work in the booming textile industry. The result is the most diverse of slums, arguably the most diverse neighborhood in Mumbai, India's most diverse city.

Stay for a while on the three-foot-wide (one meter) lane of Rajendra Prasad Chawl, and you become acquainted with the rhythms of the place. The morning sound of devotional singing is followed by the rush of water. Until recently few people in Dharavi had water hookups. Residents such as Meera Singh, a wry woman who has lived on the lane for 35 years, used to walk a mile (two kilometers) to get water for the day's cleaning and cooking. At the distant spigot she would have to pay the local "goons" to fill her buckets.

This is how it works in the bureaucratic twilight zone of informal housing. Deprived of public services because of their illegal status, slum dwellers often find themselves at the mercy of the "land mafia." There are water goons, electricity goons. In this regard, the residents of Rajendra Prasad Chawl are fortunate. These days, by DIY hook or crook, nearly every household on the street has its own water tap. And today, like every day, residents open their hoses to wash down the lane as they stand in the doorways of their homes to brush their teeth.

This is how Dharavi wakes up. On 90 Feet Road, named for its alleged width (even if 60 Feet Road, the slum's other main drag, is considerably wider), the cab drivers coax their battered Fiats to life. In the potters' neighborhood, black smoke is already pouring from six-foot-square (one square meter) kilns. By the mucky industrial canal, the recyclers are in full swing. In Dharavi nothing is considered garbage. Ruined plastic toys are tossed into massive grinders, chopped into tiny pieces, melted down into multicolored pellets, ready to be refashioned into knockoff Barbie dolls. Here every cardboard box or 55-gallon (208 liters) oil drum has another life, and another one after that.

Mornings at Rajendra Prasad Chawl are equally hectic. With the eight furniture makers to whom she rents part of her apartment gone for the day, Meera Singh combs the hair of her grandchildren: Atul, 7, Kanchan, 10, and Jyoti, 12. Soon the apartment, home to 15, is empty, save for Meera and her twenty something son, Amit, he of the dashing mustache and semi-hipster haircut. A couple of years ago, the Singh family, like everyone else in Dharavi, sat in front of the television to see local singer Abhijit Sawant win the first Indian Idol contest. But now Meera is watching her favorite TV personality, the orange-robed yoga master, Baba Ramdev, who demonstrates an anti-aging technique: rubbing your fingernails against each other at a rapid pace.

"Why listen to this fool?" dismisses Amit.

"You know nothing," Meera shoots back. "His hair is black, and he is more than 80 years old."

"Eighty? He's no more than 40. Don't fall for these cheating tricks."

Meera shakes her head. She gave up trying to talk sense to Amit long ago. "His head is in the clouds," she says. She wishes he'd get a job as did his brother Manoj, who sews jeans in one of Dharavi's *kaarkhanas*, or sweatshops. But this is not for him, Amit says. A thinker, he sees his life in terms of "a big picture." Central to this conceit is the saga of how the

Singhs came to Dharavi in the first place. Members of the *Kshatriyas,* regarded as second only to Brahmans in the caste system, Amit's great uncles were *zamindars,* or landlords, in the service of the British.

Stripped of privilege after independence, the family moved from Uttar Pradesh to Mumbai, where Amit's father worked in the textile mills. The collapse of the mills in the 1970s landed the family in Dharavi. It is this story of chance and fate ("A hundred years ago we would have been bosses," he says) that spurs Amit's outsize sense of self. He's always got a dozen things going. There's his soap powder pyramid scheme, his real estate and employment agency gambits. New is his exterminator firm, for which he has distributed hundreds of handbills ("No bedbug! No rat!"), claiming to be Dharavi's "most trusted" vermin remover, despite having yet to exterminate one cockroach.

Also on Amit's agenda is the *Janhit Times,* a tabloid he envisions as a hard-hitting advocate of grassroots democracy. The first edition featured a story about an allegedly corrupt Dharavi policeman. Amit's headline: "A Giant Bastard, a Dirty Corrupted Devil, and Uniformed Goon." Cooler heads, pointing out the policeman wielded a lethal *lathi* (bamboo nightstick), suggested a milder approach. Reluctantly Amit went with "A Fight for Justice." Even though the paper has yet to print its first edition, Amit carries a handsome press pass, which he keeps with his stack of business cards. This leads his mother to remark, "That's you, many cards, but no businesses." Looking at her son, she says, "You are such a dreamer."

It is an assessment that Amit, who just decided to open a rental car agency in hopes of diversifying his portfolio in the mode of "a Richard Branson of Dharavi," does not dispute. "Talk about doing something about Mumbai slums, and no one pays attention. Talk about Dharavi, and it is Mission Impossible, an international incident," says Mukesh Mehta as he enters the blond-paneled conference room of the Maharashtra State Administration Building. For nine years,

Mehta, a 56-year-old architect and urban designer, has honed his plan for "a sustainable, mainstreamed, slum-free Dharavi."

At today's meeting, after many PowerPoint presentations, the plan is slated for approval by the state chief minister, Vilasrao Deshmukh. Dharavi is to be divided into five sectors, each developed with the involvement of investors, mostly nonresident Indians. Initially, 57,000 Dharavi families will be resettled into high-rise housing close to their current residences. Each family is entitled to 225 square feet (21 square meters) of housing, with its own indoor plumbing. In return for erecting the "free" buildings, private firms will be given handsome incentives to build for-profit housing to be sold at (high) market rates.

"All that remains is the consent," Mehta tells Deshmukh, a sour-looking gentleman in a snow-white suit sitting with his advisers at the 40-foot (12 meters) conference table. Normally, it is required that 60 percent of Dharavi residents approve of the plan. But Deshmukh announces that formal consent is not needed because Mehta's plan is a government-sponsored project. All he must do is give the residents a month to register complaints. "A 30-day window, not a day more," Deshmukh says with impatient finality.

Later, as his driver pilots his Honda Accord through traffic, Mehta is smiling. "This is a good day," he says. "A dream comes true." At first glance, Mehta, resident of an elegant apartment building on swank Napean Sea Road, a longtime member of the British Raj era Bombay Gymkhana and Royal Bombay Yacht Club, does not appear to be a Dharavi dreamer. "You could say I was born with a golden spoon in my mouth," he remarks at his West Bandra office overlooking the Arabian Sea. "My father came to Bombay from Gujarat without a penny and built a tremendous steel business. An astrologer told him his youngest son - me - would be the most successful one, so I was afforded everything." These perks included a top education, plus a sojourn in the U.S., where Mehta studied architecture at Pratt Institute in Brooklyn.

"For me, America has always been the inspiration," says Mehta, who made a fortune managing his father's steel business before deciding to develop real estate on Long Island's exclusive North Shore. "Great Gatsby country," he says, detailing how he built high-end houses and lived in Centre Island, a white community with "the richest of the rich" such as Billy Joel, who recently listed his mansion for 37.5 million dollars.

"The slums were the furthest thing from my mind," Mehta says. This changed when he returned to Mumbai. He saw what everyone else did - that the city was filled with a few rich people, a vast number of poor people, and hardly anyone in the middle. This was most evident in the appalling housing situation. The city was split between the Manhattan-priced high-rises that dotted the south Mumbai skyline and those brownish areas on the map marked with the letters ZP for *zopadpatti*, aka slums.

Downtown business people railed that the slums were choking the life out of the city, robbing it of its rightful place in the 21st century. After all, India was no longer a post-colonial backwater famous only for the most wretched people of the Earth and the gurus who appealed to gullible Beatles. Now, when a computer broke in Des Moines, the help desk was in Bangalore. Economists were predicting exactly when the Indian GNP was likely to surpass that of the United States.

If Mumbai was going to achieve its stated destiny of becoming a world-class metropolis, a rival to China's soaring Shanghai, how could that happen when every bit of open space was covered with these eyesores, these human dumps where no one paid taxes? For Mukesh Mehta, if India were to become the ideal consumer society, it would have to develop a true middle class - and housing would be the engine. The slums would have to be reclaimed.

But which slums? There were so many of them. Then it jumped out, as clear as real estate's incontrovertible first axiom, location, location, location: Dharavi, right in the middle of the map. It was a quirk of geography and history, as any urban planner will tell you (the American inner city aside): Large masses of poor people are not supposed to be in the center of the city. They are supposed to be on the periphery, stacked up on the outskirts. Dharavi had once been on the northern fringe, but ever growing Mumbai had sprawled toward the famous slum, eventually surrounding it.

It didn't take a wizard to see the advantages of Dharavi's position. Served by two railway lines, it was ideally situated for middle-class commuters. Added to this was the advent of the Bandra-Kurla Complex, a global corporate enclave located directly across the remaining mangrove swamps, as close to Dharavi as Wall Street is to Brooklyn Heights. Sterile and kempt, the BKC was the future, right on the doorstep of the *zopadpatti*.

"I approached it as a developer. In other words, as a mercenary," says Mehta, satellite images of Dharavi spread across his desk. "But something happened. I opened an office in Dharavi, started talking to people, seeing who they were, how hard they worked, and how you could be there for months and never once be asked for a handout."

It was then, Mehta says, "I had an epiphany. I asked myself if these people were any different from my father when he first came from Gujarat. They have the same dreams. That was when I decided to dedicate the rest of my life to fixing the slums. Because I realized: The people of Dharavi - they are my genuine heroes."

Back on Rajendra Prasad Chawl, news of the plan's approval was met with a decidedly mixed response. Meera Singh barely looked up from Baba Ramdev's lecture. She had heard often the stories about Dharavi's supposed transformation. Nothing much ever happened. Why should Mukesh Mehta's scheme be any different? Moreover, what reason would possess her to move into a 225-square-foot (21 square meters) apartment, even if it were free? She has nearly 400 square feet (40 square meters). "Informal housing" has been good to her. She receives 1,100 rupees a month from the furniture workers and another thousand from renting her basement. Why should she give this up for a seven-story apartment building where she'll be saddled with fees, including "lift" charges? She doesn't like to ride in elevators. They give her the creeps.

Amit Singh was more outspoken. Mehta's plan was nothing more than "a scam, a chunk of fool's gold." Amit was already drafting an editorial in the *Janhit Times* demanding a citizen's arrest of "the gangster Mehta." In a place with one toilet for every few hundred people (the so-called politics of defecation is a perennial hot button in India), the prospect of having one's own bathroom would seem to be a powerful selling point for the plan. But even if a stir broke out last summer when gurus declared that the waters of Mahim Creek, the slum's reeking unofficial public toilet, had miraculously turned "sweet" (leading to much gastrointestinal trauma), many Dharavi locals were unmoved by the idea of a personal look.

"What need do I have of my own toilet?" asks Nagamma Shilpiri, who came to Dharavi from Andhra Pradesh 20 years ago and now lives with her crippled father and 13 other relatives in two 150-square-foot (14 square meters) rooms. Certainly, Shilpiri is embarrassed by the lack of privacy when she squats in the early morning haze beside Mahim Creek. But the idea of a personal flush toilet offends her. To use all that water for so few people seems a stupid, even sinful, waste.

Everyone in Dharavi had their own opinion about how and why the plan was concocted to hurt them in particular. The most nuanced assessment came from Shaikh Mobin, a plastics recycler in his mid-30s. Mobin has lived his whole life in Dharavi, but he'd never call himself a slum dweller. His recycling business, started by his grandfather, passed to his father, and now to him ("the post-consumer economy, turning waste into wealth," he says), had made Mobin a relatively rich man. He and his family live in a marble-floored flat at the 13-floor Diamond Apartments, "Dharavi's number one prestige address."

Mobin is a supporter of development in Dharavi. Change is necessary. Polluting industries like recycling have no business being in the center of a modern metropolis. Mobin was already making plans to move his factory several miles to the north. But this didn't mean he is happy with what is happening in the place of his birth. Much of his critique is familiar. The government's failure to create housing for middle-income people was responsible for the existence of the slums, Mobin contends.

Many people in Dharavi make enough money to live elsewhere, "a house like you see on TV." But since no such housing exists, they are doomed to the slum. Mobin doubts Mukesh Mehta's private developers will help. All over Dharavi are reminders of developmental disasters. Near Dharavi Cross Road, members of the L.P.T. Housing Society, their houses torn down in preparation for their promised apartments, have spent the past eight years living in a half-finished building without steady electricity or water, at the mercy of the goons and the malarial Mumbai heat.

But when it comes down to it, Mobin says, Dharavi's dilemma is at once much simpler and infinitely more complex: "This is our home." This is what people such as Chief Minister Deshmukh and Mukesh Mehta will never understand, Mobin says. "Mukesh Mehta says I am his hero, but what does he know of my life? He is engaged in shaikhchilli, which is dreaming, dreaming in the day. Does it occur to him that we do not wish to be part of his dream?"

Such sentiments cause Mukesh Mehta distress. "If someone calls me a dreamer, I plead guilty," he says, finishing his crème caramel at the Bombay Yacht Club. To be sure, Mehta has made some fanciful statements regarding Dharavi's future. His idea to install a golf driving range has met with widespread guffaws. "Golf? What is this golf?" asked Shilpiri's crippled father. The other day Mehta was fantasizing about constructing a 120,000-seat cricket stadium in the slum. Asked where fans would park, Mehta looked stricken.

"Parking! Oh, my God," he exclaimed. "I'm going to be up all night trying to figure that out."

But being a dreamer doesn't mean he is "unrealistic," Mehta says. He has been around the block of India's bruising bureaucracy. He has learned hard lessons along the way. One is that "sometimes the last thing people in power want is to get rid of slums." Much of what Mehta calls "slum perpetuation" has to do with the infamous "vote bank" - a political party through a deep-rooted system of graft, lays claim to the vote of a particular neighborhood. As long as the slum keeps voting the right way, it's to the party's advantage to keep the community intact.

A settlement can remain in the same place for years, shelters passing from makeshift plastic tarps to corrugated metal to concrete. But one day, as in the case of Dharavi, the slum might find itself suddenly in the "wrong" place. Once that happens, the bulldozer is always a potential final solution. A few years ago, the Maharashtra government, under the direction of Chief Minister Deshmukh, in a spasm of upgrading supposedly aimed at closing the "world-class" gap, demolished 60,000 hutments, some in place for decades. As many as 300,000 people were displaced.

This, Mehta says, is what his plan is devised to avoid. "No one wants to be that unhappy guy driving the bulldozer." Preferring "the talking cure," Mehta says if anyone, anywhere, doesn't think his plan is the best possible outcome for Dharavi, he will sit with them for as long as it takes, to convince them. A few days later, at Kumbharwada, he got his chance.

To many, the Kumbhar potters are the heart and soul of Dharavi. Their special status derives not only from their decades-long residence but also from the integrity of their work. While Dharavi is famous for making use of things everyone throws away, the Kumbhars create the new.

Savdas family members have been Dharavi potters for generations, but Tank Ranchhod Savdas once imagined another kind of life. "I had big dreams," he says. "I thought I would be a lawyer." But Tank's father died in 1986, and "as the oldest son I took up this business." Not that he has any regrets. "During busy times, I make hundreds of pots a day, and I get pleasure from each one," he says.

Recently, however, the fortyish "Mr. Tank" has begun to fear for the future of *Kumbhars* in Dharavi. Increasing numbers of the community's young men have become merchant seamen, or computer specialists at the Bandra-Kurla Complex. Kumbharwada is full of teenage boys who have never used a potter's wheel, unthinkable only a few years ago.

And now there is this plan. Just talking about "a slum-free Dharavi" is enough to make Tank shake with anger. How dare anyone claim that Kumbharwada is "a slum" in need of rehabilitation! Kumbharwada is home to working people, men and women who have always made their own way. If Mukesh Mehta was so enamored of the U.S., couldn't he see Kumbharwada was a sterling example of the supposed American dream?

"Look at my house," Tank demands, showing off the 3,000-square-foot (280 square meters) home and workshop he built and now shares with his two brothers and their families. "Why should we move from here, to there?"

By "there," Tank means the Slum Rehabilitation Authority high-rise under construction behind Kumbharwada. Freshly painted, the building has a sprightly look, but soon lack of maintenance will turn it into a replica of every other SRA building: a decaying Stalinist-styled pile, covered with Rorschach-like mildew stains. Inside is a long, dank hallway with 18 apartments on either side, which Amit Singh calls "36 rooms of gloom."

"That is a slum," says Tank, "a vertical slum." Told that Mehta says he's willing to talk with anyone unhappy with the plan, Tank says, "Then bring him here. Tomorrow."

On his cell phone from Hyderabad, Mehta, "not risk averse," says "ten o'clock." But he is skeptical the meeting will accomplish much. He's spoken with the potters many times. Proposals allowing them to keep the majority of their space have been rejected, as was his idea to maximize the potters' profits by adding ornamental ceramics to their traditional vessels and religious objects. "I've offered them the moon and been repaid with crushing indifference," Mehta bemoans. Plus, he never knows which alleged leadership group represents whom.

It's a frustrating situation that one afternoon causes the Americanized Mehta to shout, "Your trouble is you have too many chiefs and not enough Indians!" Yet when ten o'clock rolls around, there he is, impeccably attired in a tan suit, cuff links gleaming in the sunlight, in the courtyard in front of Tank's house. Perhaps a hundred people have assembled, sitting on plastic chairs. Most are potters, but there are others, too, such as Amit Singh and several colleagues from the Janhit Times. After politely listening to Mehta's short form of the plan (he has brought his PowerPoint presentation, but sunlight prevents its deployment), the objections begin.

It is outrageous that this was even being discussed, people say. "We have been making pots for 130 years," one man shouts. "This land is ours." Mehta is sympathetic to the Kumbhar position. But there are a few "realities" they must understand. First, the assumption that the community owns the Kumbharwada grounds by virtue of the British Raj-era Vacant Land Tenancy act is incorrect. Mehta says the *Kumbhars'* long-term lease ran out when the act was repealed in 1974. Also, there is the pollution issue. Every day the potters' brick kilns send huge black clouds into the air. It's gotten so bad that nearby Sion Hospital is complaining that the smoke is aggravating patients' pulmonary ailments.

The Kumbhars are vulnerable on these issues, Mehta says. Chief Minister Deshmukh would be within his rights to send the dreaded bulldozers rolling down 90 Feet Road. The *Kumbhars* should trust him, Mehta says. His very presence proves his sincerity. "People said if I came here, I should wear a hard hat. But you see me, bareheaded." At the very least, the *Kumbhars* should allow him to conduct a census of the area.

This information would help him fight for them, get them the best deal.

With the return of the late monsoon rains, the session breaks up. Mehta gets back into his chauffeured car feeling upbeat. "A good meeting," he says. The fact that the *Kumbhars* seemed to agree to the census was a good sign, Mehta says, driving off through puddles. Back at Kumbharwada, Tank is asked what he has learned from the meeting. Surrounded by perhaps 20 potters, Tank says, "We have learned that Mukesh Mehta's plan is of no use to us." Would they participate in the census? "We'll think about it," says Tank.

In any event, there is no time to talk about it now. The meeting has taken almost two hours. With orders piling up, there is work to be done. Mukesh Mehta's plan is scheduled to be implemented sometime this year, not that Dharavi is excessively fixated on it during holiday season, a time to, as a sign in the window of Jayanthian fireworks store on 90 Feet Road says, "enjoy the festivals with an atom bomb." Today is Ganesh Chaturthi, and much of Dharavi (the Hindus, anyway) are in the streets beating giant drums and blaring Bollywood-inflected songs on car-battery-powered speakers in celebration of Lord Ganesh. Ganesh, the roly-poly elephant god, has special significance in Dharavi, being considered the deity of "removing obstacles."

One such obstacle is in evidence at the outset of the parade marking the end of the ten-day festival for which people make giant *murtis*, or likenesses, of the god. These effigies are borne through the streets to Mahim Beach and then tossed into the water. One group has constructed a ten-foot-high (three meters) Ganesh from silvery papier-mâché. They have not, however, bothered to measure the narrow lane through which the Ganesh will need to pass to reach Dharavi Main Road.

After much discussion and a tortuous 50-foot (15 meters) journey during which many Dharavian "obstacles," including a ganglia of illegally connected electric wires, needed to be removed, the murti makes it through with a quarter inch to spare. Not a bit of the god's silvery skin is nicked. As the

Ganesh is lifted onto a flatbed truck for its journey to Mahim Beach, one resident turns and says, "You see. The Ganesh is undamaged. This is our talent. We deal with what is."

SLUM LITERACY IN INDIA

Disparity means unequal possession of particular property or attributes between two or more social groups or regions. Inequality means that certain individuals or groups in a society are in a relatively disadvantageous situation in regard to the access to and possession of various societal resources including literacy/education. Literacy has been considered one of the most important attributes for social development. It is seen as a prerequisite for economic growth, social mobility and political stability. Illiteracy, by contrast, has frequently been related to increased poverty, under development, political volatility and economic stagnation.

In terms of literacy there is marked regional variation as well as different level of literacy between social groups has been observed. Education is also viewed as important for achieving economic development and technical progress, crucial for social transformation towards a better order based on values of freedom, social justice an equal opportunity. Slums have become worldwide phenomena in urban areas and 31.6 of the world urban population live in slums. The slum dwellers belong to among one of the poorest section of the urban society. In India, 15 percent of total urban population has no option but to get their shelter in slums.

Marked disparity is also observed with regard to literacy level between non-slum dwellers and slum dwellers in many part of India. Slums are physical and spatial manifestation of increasing urban poverty and intra-city inequality. However, slums do not accommodate all of the urban poor, nor are all slum dwellers always poor. Although the term 'slum' is considered an easily understandable catchall, it disguises the fact that within this and other terms lie a multitude of different settlements and communities. The major urban concern is the growing gap between the demand and supply of basic infrastructure services like safe drinking water, sanitation, sewerage, housing, energy, transport, communication, health and education.

Increased Urbanisation adversely affects the quality of life of the people some times and many times it leads to negligence of education for economically deprived section of the society especially in the slums and squatter settlement. The Millennium Development Goals (MDGs) play an important role in making strategy for reduction of world disparity. Broadly, the MDGs aim to reduce global poverty, improve the lives of the poor and increase the pace of development in a sustainable manner. Many of the goal, target and indicator has direct link with slum education. Goal 2 focuses on Universal Primary Education, which ensures that all boys and girls should complete a full course of primary schooling. Goal 3 is also relevant with reference to slum education and it stands for elimination of gender disparity in primary and secondary education, preferably by 2005, and in all levels of education no later than 2015.

Goal 7: Target 11 gives attention on the issue of slums and the improvement of the lives of the slum dwellers. However, in order to face the challenges of the slum dwellers, one needs to be considering the other facet of the problem through goals and target and given indicators. The condition of slum will not improve in if nothing can be done to achieve other goals in integrated manner. The human development index (HDI) developed by United Nations Development Program (UNDP) is often regarded as an alternative to income-based measures of welfare.

HDI has three indicators: Longevity, Education and Standard of living. It shows that rising income is not the only central concern of human development, but education and literacy are also important for development of nation and society. Literacy creates the conditions for stimulating initiatives as well as human participation in creation of projects that act upon, transform the world and define the aims and objectives of an authentic human development. Literacy has been defined differently by different sources. According to definition given by dictionary, literacy refers to capacity to read and write with certain level of education. Literacy is normally considered in terms of both reading and writing with understanding. In India right from the beginning of the census in 1872, literates were enumerated and literacy rates were calculated. From 1961 onwards children of the age 4 or less were not treated even if they had picked up reading and writing a few odd words. Only a person who had attained the age 5 was considered literate.

In the 1991 census this age has been raised up to 7 as the Department of Education of the Ministry of Human Resource Development and the Planning Commission felt that the ability to read and write with understanding is not ordinarily achieved especially in many backward areas, until one had some schooling or had at least some time to develop skills. However, the way literacy gets defined the fact remains that because of historical, social and economic reasons different regions not only have different level of literacy, but there may be disparate levels of literacy attainment between various social groups, locations and gender within a region.

The study aims at building up of a literacy scenario of slums. An attempt has been done to trace the spatial pattern of literacy for slums and non-slum population and to measure disparities in literacy therein. This study is based on acceptance of basic differences in a given society between 'have' and 'have not' and argues that any disparities by themselves are not as meaningful as when compared to what can be termed as 'reference group'. Equity can be examined only by the actual distribution of different socio- economic phenomenon against certain normative distribution, the latter reflecting the value judgment of the community in the context of a given set of development objectives. Disparity index has been calculated by the formula suggested by Kundu and Rao, which is in fact, modified version of Sopher's Index for measurement for disparity.

The database for the study has been taken from Census of India 2001 results. Size class distribution of the disparity index across the region has been done statistically where mean and standard deviation are taken as the basis of categorization for every variable and for each study unit. Hence, the real value of one category of disparity is not equal to real value another category of disparity. The paper has been organized into five sections. First section deals with introduction of the topic whereas Conclusion and policy implication deals with last section. Section two explains general picture of incidence of slum and Urbanisation in India. General scenario of slum and non-slum literacy has been incorporated in section three at state and million plus city level. Section four describes pattern of disparity in slum education.

SLUMS AND URBANISATION

Generally, a slum is defines as a compact settlement with a collection of poorly built tenements, mostly of temporary nature, crowded together usually with inadequate and drinking water facilitates in unhygienic conditions. An area is considered as "non-notified slum" if at least 20 households lived in that area. Areas notified as slums by respective municipalities, corporations, local bodies or developmental authorities are treated as "notified slum". Much of the data on urban poverty focuses on slums. Slums are mainly urban phenomena where poverty gets clustered. One out every seven person living in the urban areas lives in the slums of India.

The figure goes up when we consider it for towns reporting slums and 23.6 percent population of the slum reporting towns' lives in the slums. Meghalaya have shown exceptionally high incidence of slum i.e. 65 percent of the slum reporting towns. Some the states like Haryana, Chhattisgarh Madhya Pradesh, Maharastra and Andhra Pradesh have shown very high incidence of slum than the national average. Do all urban centers of India have slum? No only 640 out of 5161 urban areas have reported slums. It means only 12.7 percent of total Indian towns have reported slum. The distribution of these towns across the states and union territories is not uniform.

Andhra Pradesh had highest number of towns having slum i.e. 77. In other words, 36 percent towns of this state have reported slum. Chandigarh, on the other hand, have slum in all census towns. Only few states have shown have less slum-reporting towns than national average. They are Punjab, Haryana, Bihar, West Bengal, Chhatisgarh, Maharashtra, Karnataka and Andhra Pradesh. The comparison between concentration of urban population and incidence of slums across the states gives a clear understanding that only few states accommodates larger population of slum dwellers. Maharatra, Andhra Pradesh, Tamil Nadu, Madhya Pradesh, Uttar Pradesh and Delhi together have more than 66 percent slum dwellers of India. Is level of Urbanisation closely associated with incidences of slum in majority of the Indian states?

A large number of states experiencing high percentage of slums to urban population are also showing high level of Urbanisation (e. g. Punjab, Haryana, West Bengal and Maharastra) where as the situation is not same if both incidence of slum and level of Urbanisation is low (Bihar and Assam) Rajasthan emerged as the only state where both are moderate. Gujarat, Kerala and Karnataka have high level of Urbanisation but incidence of slum is comparatively low. Hence, high level of Urbanisation does not mean better well being because many times it leads to high incidence of slums. Slums and Urbanisation are the two extreme phenomena, which may exist together or not. Development of slum cannot be said as a desirable incident. In India, Slums are not present in every urban center but they have significant role in the development.

LITERACY SCENARIO IN SLUMS OF INDIA

Urban area does not mean very high literacy and well developed all the time. The intra city disparity exists everywhere though the degree is not uniform. In general, the level of literacy in slums area has been found less than the non-slum areas. Regional variations in the distribution of male literacy exist in every state. Tripura and Meghalaya reported more than 80 percents literate males whereas males residing in the slums of Delhi and Chandigarh are at the bottoms were the level of slum literacy is 43 and 55 respectively. Kerala and Maharashtra observed very high male literacy but Karnataka, Bihar and Uttar Pradesh do not have satisfactory male literacy in the slum areas. The condition of women in the slums appears to be more critical. The level of female slum literacy has been observed around 55 percent for the all India level. It has been found lowest in Chandigarh i.e. 30 per cent and highest 75.5 percent in Meghalaya.

Female slum literacy in some of the states like Jammu and Kashmir, Delhi, Rajasthan, Uttar Pradesh, Gujarat and Goa are far below than the national average. Non-slum areas emerge at better stage and majority of the states have more than 65 percent literate population. In case of male literacy for non-slums area all India figure is 76 percent whereas it comes down to 65 percent in Uttar Pradesh and goes up to 85 percent for Kerala and Tripura. Kerala emerged as the only state where there is very high literacy rate for female in non-slum areas i.e. 84 percent while national average is only 65 percent. Almost all the educationally backward state showed low literacy for non-slum areas.

Below, Incidence of slum and status of literacy level in Municipal Corporation having population having more than one million has been analyzed. Greater Mumbai accommodates largest slum dwellers and 48 percent of its population lives in slums. Patna has only 0.25 percent populations living in slums whereas Lucknow, on other hand, has reported no slum at all. Some of the municipal corporation, which shows high incidence of slums, is Kolkata, Nagpur, Thane, Meerut and Faridabad. Low incidence of slum has been found in Bangalore, Bhopal, Vadodara, Agra and Kalyan Municipal Corporation.. It means, the population size of the municipal corporation have no significant relation ship with incidence of slums. Similarly, the status of literacy level in these cities shows high diversity.

Slums of Nagpur show highest literacy level where the literacy rates are 80, 69 and 75 for male, female and person category respectively. The situation becomes reverse in case of Patna and it is at the bottom in every category. Jaipur slums have only half of the population having ability to read and write. The situation for female slum dwellers is worse here where only 39 percent females are literate. The situation is different across these cities for non-slum literacy. A large number of cities concentrated around 80 percent male literacy. In Greater Mumbai and Chennai, the literacy level for male and female is highest i.e. 85 percent. Lowest literacy of around 67 percent has been observed for Agra and Varanasi Municipal Corporation. It becomes clear from the above analysis, marked disparity has been observed with regard to literacy level between non-slum dwellers and slum dwellers in many part of India and the level of literacy for female living in the slum experience educational deprivation.

GENDER LITERACY IN THE SLUM

The slum dwellers belong to the poorest section of the urban society. Women constitute half of the human population, yet their position in society is secondary to men and this is by and large true for the majority of communities. Significant disparity between male and female has also been noticed. Here we have calculated disparity between slum non-slum male disparity, slum non-slum female disparity, slum non-slum disparity in literacy and gender disparity within slums at different levels. Meghalaya emerged as the only state where male slum non-slum disparity has been found reverse. It is the non-slum area that has lees male literacy than the slum areas.

Tripura showed lowest male slum non-slum disparity where the gap between the literacy levels is marginal. Punjab, Uttar Pradesh, Jharkhand, Chhattisgarh, Madhya Pradesh, Maharashtra and Tamil Nadu observed less slum non-slum male literacy than the national average i.e. 6.52. The situation becomes worse for Chandigarh where the gap between Slum and non- slum literacy goes up to 25 percent. Even Kerala, which is known for better literacy status, has comparatively high disparity for males residing in slums. In case of female literacy gap between slum and non-slum areas all India shows high figure of 10 percent. Meghalaya once again has same reverse disparity. Tripura also had same status. Slums of Jharkhand have reported less disparity in female literacy between slum and non-slum areas.

Jammu and Kashmir, Punjab, Uttar Pradesh, Madhya Pradesh and Tamil Nadu are other states, which had less female slum non-slum disparity in literacy. Chandigarh and Goa showed very gap in female literacy between slum and non-slum areas and the corresponding figures are 42 and 33 percent respectively. Overall disparity in literacy between slum and non-slum areas is 8 percent and this figure is not uniform across the states. We have few states, which do not show disparity in education between slum and non-slum area in urban centers. Some of the educationally backward states like Uttar Pradesh and Madhya Pradesh do not show much difference in the levels of literacy between slum and non-slums. Similarly, Tamil Nadu where the level of literacy is high does not area specific disparity in literacy.

On the other hand, Chandigarh, Delhi, Gujarat, Rajasthan and Karnataka experience very high disparity in literacy for slum area. Interestingly, Kerala also shows significant disparity in spite of the fact that she has very high literacy level. At last, it appears that there is no relationship between general level of literacy and disparity between slum and non-slum literacy. The pattern of disparity in literacy emerges tells different story for male and female. We have one category of states like Tamil Nadu and Meghalaya where low disparity in literacy in the entire category between slum and non-slum areas and general level of literacy is high.

There emerges another pattern, where the general level of literacy is high but and has also high slum and non- slum disparity in literacy e.g. Kerala and Uttranchal. Third pattern comes out here is the states having low literacy level and having negligible slum and non slum disparity (Madhya Pradesh and Jharkhand). The behaviour of cities in terms of disparity in literacy is highly uneven. The slum of cities like Indore, Varanasi and Ludhiana are not much deprived in terms of literacy for both male and female. On the other extreme, Kalyan-Dombivli, Delhi and Patna observed very high disparity in literacy. It is also evident that female are the vulnerable group, because large number of cites were found clustered in the category of high or very high disparity level. Gender disparity is concerned with male-female disparity for slum dwellers and non-slum dwellers separately.

No nation can progress neglecting female education. Both the Gender related Development Index (GDI) and Capability Poverty Measures (CPM), as developed by UNDP have literacy as a key component because women's education as a multiplier effect on family well being and development of society (Mukherjee 1996) Phadke (1967, Madhav (1973) and Visarai (1993) opine that attitude of male and parents towards the education of girls and the kind of domestic work deliberately assigned to them are the reason which have kept females away from attaining education which ultimately caused low level of literacy among.

Low gender disparity within slum and high slum non-slum female disparity in literacy has been noticed in Punjab, Kerala and Karnataka. Some of the economically developed administrative units like Gujarat, Chandigarh and Goa indicate that how slum women has been ignored and they are educationally deprived. Majority of Indian experience gender disparity within slum is more visible than slum non- slum female disparity. The over picture comes out from the above analysis states that the educational status of female living in the slum is not up to mark and is facing significant gender disparity within slum.

INTRA-CITY DISPARITY IN LITERACY AMONG THE SLUM REPORTING MUNICIPAL WARDS

Urban poverty is becoming a severe, pervasive - and largely unacknowledged - feature of urban life. Large sections of the population in urban areas are suffering from extreme deprivation that is often even more debilitating than that experienced by the rural poor. The above graph shows spatial distribution of slum across the municipal ward. In the first category, we have Metro cities like Kolkata and Delhi, where around 80 percent administrative units have reported slum but percentage of slum dwellers to urban population in the city is not same.

The mega city like Ahmedabad and Jaipur, slums are also located in most of the wards but population pressure of the slum dweller for city is less. Comparatively, smaller million plus cites (Indore and Ludhiana) show agglomeration effect, here slum are located in few localities with high population pressure In the cities like Delhi and Kolkata the incidence of slum are fairly high but distribution of these slum in the city is not uniform. Slums are visible everywhere in Kolkata where 95 percent of municipal ward reported slum. In Delhi, 18 percent population lives in slum and only 67 percent of municipal ward reported slum. Level of slum literacy in Delhi shows major rift between the municipal wards having highest and lowest slum literacy level. This gap is very high and its value is more than 70 percent.

In case of non-slum, the story is totally different. Here the literacy gap is around 30 percent. It means, the slums of Delhi are not uniform in terms of level of literacy. Slums are very poor in educational attainment and there exist wide disparities between slum and non-slum literacy in Delhi. In Kolkata the range of literacy slum across the wards are 46%, 75% and 72% male, female and person respectively. But in non-slum areas this gap of literacy across the wards comes down to 18 percent, 30 percent and 24 percent for male, female and person are respectively. Ahmedabad and Jaipur are the cities where total population of the cities varies in between 20 million and 50 million and incidence of slum is less than 15 percent. The level of slum male literacy varies from 75 to 35 percent and females literacy from 20 to 64 percent across the municipal wards of Ahmedabad.

In the municipal wards of Jaipur slums, the range of male literacy varies from 86 to 43 percent and female literacy from

69 to 20 percent. Indore and Ludhiana are among one the important industrial cities of India. The incidences of slums in these cities are 16.2 and 22.5 percent respectively. These two cities have better slum literacy because they have minimum gap between slum and non-slum literacy. More than 50 percent, males residing in the slum are literate in these two cities. In case of female slum literacy, it is Indore where the females are more literate among the all selected cities. Non-slum areas of these two cities have almost similar pattern of male and female literacy. Now the question comes, is level of disparity in slum literacy uniformly distributed within the city.

Slum non-slum male disparity in literacy have almost similar pattern of distribution in Kolkata and Delhi. The distribution seems to more normal in case of Kolkata and around 80 percent municipal wards low to medium disparity with respect to their corresponding city. Intra city slum non-slum disparity in female literacy in between these cities has entirely different story. In Delhi, more than 42 percent slum reporting wards have low or very low level of slum non- slum female disparity in literacy where as 58 percent of the wards of Kolkata have low disparity. The distribution of gender disparity in literacy within slum of Delhi and Kolkata observe entirely different pattern. In Delhi, 17 percent slums have very low gender disparity; it means nothing much difference in terms of male and female literacy.

Similarly more than 17 percent slum reporting wards or Delhi have high of very high disparity, which shows gap of literacy level of male and female is very high. Kolkata do not report these extreme cases. Slum non-slum disparity in literacy across the municipal wards is more or less similar pattern in Ahmedabad. At the both extremes of high and very low category, the concentration in less. It means a little less than half of the wards reporting slum have medium to high level of disparity. In Jaipur the situation gets change. Comparatively larger numbers of wards have very low disparity and it is even higher in case of female. Around 47 percent of the wards having slums in this city experience medium to high disparity in literacy the non slum areas. The distribution of gender disparity in literacy in slum reporting wards of Ahmedabad indicates no uniformity of literacy among the wards.

At the one end we have 10 per cent municipal wards with very low gender disparity; on the other hand there are 7.5 percent wards with very high gender literacy. Jaipur slums have more uniformity because majority of slums of the city have middle level of disparity. The comparison of distribution of level of disparity between Ludhiana and Indore cities states that these cities are not similar. Slum non-slum disparity in male and female literacy has been found distributed distribution of in all the category in Ludhiana where as no slum of the Indore have very high slum non slum disparity in male and female literacy.

The overall condition of slum women in Indore seems to worse than non slum women in Indore. Gender disparity in literacy within slum again states that the disparity is high or very high for more than 15 percent slums in Indore while it comes down to nearly 7 percent for Ludhiana. Similarly around 80 percent slum of Ludhiana expertise low or very low gender disparity whereas 48 percent slums of Indore have same level of disparity. Rank correlation between slum non-slum male literacy gap and slum non-slum female literacy gap is very high and significant everywhere except in Ludhiana where it is significant but strength of relationship is moderate. It indicates that male and female disparity in literacy between slum and non-slum area exists together. Nothing much difference has been observed for rank correlation between slum non-slum male literacy gap and slum non-slum person literacy.

The situation is almost similar for rank correlation between slum non-slum female literacy gap and slum non-slum person literacy. Gender disparity within slum and slum non-slum male disparity do not go side by side. In many cases, if gender disparity exists then it is not necessary that there will be high and slum non-slum male disparity in literacy. Moderate and significant relationship between gender disparity within slum and slum non-slum female disparity has been found in every case except Ahmedabad and Jaipur. It gives clear indication that the condition of female in not desirable in both the places slum as well as in non-slum areas. The impact of gender disparity within slum gives similar results for correlation between gender disparity within slum and slum non-slum person disparity.

A major locational disparity in literacy between slum and non-slum emerge out from the analysis. Similarly gender discrimination in literacy still appears to a major issue. Female literacy does show their critical condition not only in slum but also outside the slum in the city. In sum it has been observed in the study that literacy level of slum dwellers, particularly female literacy is extremely low in comparison to non-slum dwellers population, the gender disparity for slum dwellers is markedly higher than non-slum dwellers gender disparity. It is true that Universal Elementary Education (UEE) has become a popular slogan but do we have any honest effort to achieve this goal for the people in living in the slums.

The government sponsored either on going or previous programme like National Slum Development Programme. Sarva Siksha Abhiyan (SSA), National Literacy Mission (NLM), Integrated Child Development Programme (ICDS) have never given special attention to the slum education. Still, we have Jawaharlal Nehru National Urban Renewal Mission (JLNURM), but what is happening with slum education? Proving elementary education to slum dwellers is not the part of the mission. Do providing basic services to Urban Poor do not need education? Do we have enough educational infrastructures in the slum or we have achieved universal elementary education in the slums?

It is clear from the status of slums literacy that Slum Education has remained an ignorant sector of human resource planning in India. What is needed is the location specific educational development programme and planning with focus on the slums having very low literacy level and high gender disparity in literacy. Target area should be the focus of planning since slum does not represent common society. Slums are physical manifestation of urban poverty, where child labour is easily visible; mainly informal sector of employment exist; have no or very poor basic services like housing, water and electricity; Immigration is prevalent; and mass illiteracy and gender discrimination is present. In these circumstances how it is possible for a poor bread earner to sent their children in the schools, which are present outside the slum. Slums require special schools where learning and earning can coexist.

10

Slum Culture in Bangladesh

HEALTH AND SOCIAL CONDITIONS IN THE DHAKA SLUMS

Homelessness and poverty are an international crisis. Bangladesh, with a population of 147.4 million is one of the poorest countries in the world; with an estimated 3.4 million people live in some 5000 slums of its capital city, Dhaka. In 2010, the population of the city of Dhaka has been projected at 17.6 million people, with up to 60% in the slums. Slums, which are heavily populated urban areas characterized by poverty and substandard housing, are not well described in the literature despite their prevalence and the pervasiveness of poverty world wide. The last study of the urban poor was the 1995 Survey of Urban Poverty in Bangladesh.

The Bangladesh Demographic and Health Survey (BDHS) is a periodic study of the population and although urban areas are surveyed, slums are not specifically investigated. Urban planning to accommodate increasingly large slum areas requires study to determine demographics and determinants of improved quality of life, such as health status, health services, financial stability, education and security. In this pilot study, we describe 100 families living in Dhaka slum areas. Migration, living conditions, social structure, child and adult health and health care, income, nutrition, and contraceptive practices are examined. Comparison is made to the Survey of Urban Poverty in Bangladesh, the BDHS, and to existing literature. Potential areas to target for intervention are also explored.

METHODS

We undertook a 115-question survey, of a convenience sample of 100 heads of household living in 3 slum areas of Dhaka. The questions were based on a survey administered to the homeless in Ottawa (the Ottawa Population Health Survey), were adjusted to be culturally sensitive and were translated to Bengali. The study was approved by the Ottawa Hospital research ethics board. Questions were mainly closed-ended.

Eight surveyors were trained and the survey field-tested prior to general administration. Inclusion criteria required subject age over 20 and residence in the slum for more than one year. A consent and confidentiality statement was read aloud, and the interview conducted with subject consent. Interviews took place from April-July 2002. Respondents were paid 300 Taka per interview and given a bucket to collect fresh water for participation. Interviews were conducted in one sitting.

RESULTS

A sample of 100 subjects was recruited from the Mohammadpur (n= 41), Lalbagh (n=12) and Dhanmondi (n=47) slums of Dhaka, Bangladesh. Twelve were male and 88 were female with an average age of 35 years. Subjects were mostly married and were associated with 84 spouses; the majority (81%) had received no schooling.

They had 296 children (3.1 ± 1.5 children per family) and 31 other dependents (in-laws and siblings) living with them, thus a total of 511 people are represented in the results. Of the 96 married subjects, 84 lived with their spouse; three husbands lived closer to work, and seven women reported their husbands to be polygamous, living with a second wife. Most families (45%) had been living in the current slum for less than two years.

Migration

The majority (93%) of the subjects were born in outside villages, an average of 255 km from the slum. Most described an economic migration, citing poverty (76%), inability to find work (29%) and sell-off of their land (27%) as reasons they left the countryside. A further 19% described family conflict or violence, and 21% cited floods or land erosion. Eighty families had been living in another slum prior to the current and reasons cited for moving were eviction (27), rent increase (15), lack of drinking water (4), dirty environment (5), threat to personal safety (9), loss of job (2), fire (4), and flood (1).

Living Conditions

Slum land was owned by a landowner or *basti* (slum) owner for 83%, and rent collected for permission to build a bamboo shelter to use as a home. Landowners and *basti* owners are not thought to pay government taxes and are not accountable for the conditions or safety of the slums. Government land is also illegally occupied by so-called "musclemen," who build slum dwellings or rent bare land plots, and allegedly maintain corrupt links with police and political parties; the remainder lived on these lands. On top of rent and the cost of security paid to the landowners and muscle men, the subjects were variably charged for the use of facilities such as toilet (46%), drinking water (87%), bathing water (13%), electricity (78%) and gas (6%).

All families lived in one-room dwellings, with construction usually of bamboo frame, fencing and roof. Forty-five of 100 dwellings were built elevated over water. An average of 5 people lived in each room, and four families had over eight individuals in one room. Drinking water was from a tube well for most, and five to 100+ families shared each well. The rest used city tap water, also sharing one tap among many. A latrine area (pit or elevated) was located outside the room for most (86%). The rest used a lake, river or non- designated latrine areas as a toilet. Bathing water was from a tube well, standing water or river water, and subjects bathed themselves and their children daily, and their clothes 2-7 times per week. Electricity was available to 84 of the families, though only 34 had electricity in their rooms. Nineteen of the 84 reported paying bills to the company; the other 65 splice the wire illegally, and paid the slumlord. Mud stoves were hand made and wood purchased by 94% for meal preparation; most cooked their meals in or just outside their homes.

Most respondents (89%) did not feel that they lived in a hygienic environment, and 93% felt that the slum had lead to disease or ill health in their families. The most desirable place to live was felt to be in their village of origin (57%), while others dreamed of living in higher-class places in the city (14%), a place more quiet (14%) or free of mosquitoes (5%).

Only 6% were happy in their current location. Evils described were unclean latrine facilities (30%), harassment by slum owners and the need to pay bribes (10%), lack of employment (32%), mosquitoes (86%), extremes of heat (5%), leaking roof (11%), harassment of women (7%) lack of available fuel/gas (17%) and lack of food (3%). Barriers preventing a move to a more desirable location were stated as a lack of funds (91%), lack of land (11%), inability to find work (10%), lack of government assistance (14%), illiteracy (2%) and large family size (1%). Most felt that they would not attain a better standard of life without government assistance, though 57% reported trying to save their own money to this end.

Support desired from the government included land (80%), subsidized homes (31%) and jobs (9%) with a few hoping for a rickshaw, or a bull to plough the land. From NGOs they hoped for loans (77%) land (18%), educational facilities (17%), medical treatment facilities (12%), ready-made houses (7%) and food (1%). NGOs provided some support for 24 of the families; 15 had schooling for 19 children, 7 were receiving micro credit and 2 received cooperative assistance.

Children There were 3.1 ± 1.5 children per family, average age 10 years 2 months. Only 27 of 228 school-aged children had attended school, 16 higher than primary school. A further 43 could read, 42 could read and write and 8 attended non-formal schooling. Children who worked to help support the household (n=35) were generally unable to attend school.

Children's health was reported to be good to very good (76%) while 19% noted it was poor. Reasons for poor health included rheumatic fever (3), tuberculosis (2), leprosy (1), abscess (4), epilepsy (4), disabled hand or leg (4), kidney disease (1) and non-specific descriptions (5). Immunization ("with the six major" diphtheria, pertussis, tetanus, measles, poliomyelitis, tuberculosis) was reported by 89% surveyed, and 89% reported their children received vitamin A. Fifty-eight families had one or more children die, reporting a total of 89 deaths with 50 (56%) dying before 1 year old. While diarrhea, respiratory disease, trauma and stillbirth were cited as known causes, a far greater number did not know the cause of their child's death.

Forty-two of 58 respondents sought treatment before the death of their child, while 16 were not able to consult a health care worker due to poverty (7) and lack of time (2); the remainder (7) were unable to answer. Total death rates were not calculable as the children were counted per household and not per family.

Adult Health Physical disabilities of the interviewees were enumerated; vision or hearing loss was reported by 5, handicapped hand or leg in 5, and chronic back pain in 2; these disabilities were severe enough to limit daily activities. Common chronic conditions included headaches, arthritis, back pain and urinary incontinence. Pain prevented 19 from performing most activities. Acute/recent conditions were typically jaundice, worms, joint pain, and sexually transmitted disease. Symptoms of visual impairment were reported: 23 were farsighted (hyperopic) and 17 were nearsighted (myopic), with 20 able to obtain corrective glasses.

In self-report, 9 noted cataracts and 31 had glaucoma. Hearing difficulties were noted by 24%. Five people reported needing the help of another person to walk, and another 12 required a cane. Memory was appraised and 24% responded that they were unable to remember anything/most things, and 54% remembered most things. It was not felt to be culturally sensitive to ask questions regarding psychosis, depression or suicide. Injuries and accidents were reported by 47% in the past year. These included cuts, concussions, poisoning, assault, motor vehicle accidents, and accidents involving machinery. Dental health was reported as poor or very poor in 20 and 58 reported problems with their mouth or gums. Eleven had received dental services in the past year, and 30 had 1-6 missing teeth.

Health Facilities

Health care providers were sought by 61 respondents in the past 6 months; a doctor by 44, a homeopath by 4, a "quack" (traditional medicine) by 3 and NGO clinics by 16. Twenty-five respondents were taking medicine, and 62 had prescriptions but were not taking medication due to cost. When asked if their families receive the health services that they need, 67 did "sometimes," and 32 responded "never." Health care facilities were government- run, NGO-run and private. Facilities charged for services, and a third each felt that the charges were expensive, moderate and low. Subjects were asked what they would be willing to pay for services. Most felt that immunization, contraceptive services and consultation should be free, but were willing to pay 5-20 Taka for children's care and antenatal checkups. Children were born at home, and were very occasionally delivered by trained birth attendants (5 of 296 deliveries) or in a hospital (6 deliveries). Mothers frequently returned to their home land for delivery (150 births) or delivered at home in the slum attended by elder family members (135).

Nutrition

Rice and vegetables were consumed daily by all but foods with higher protein content were consumed daily by less than 20%. Meals were consumed three times per day in 89% of families.

When asked: "Do you feel that your family eats a balanced diet and receives proper nutrition?" 94% responded negatively.

Subjects were asked if they or their family ever go hungry; 90% responded "sometimes" and 10% said "never."

Reproductive Health

Contraception was used by 64%. Methods are cited. Reasons for not using contraception as well as hygiene during the menstrual cycle were also noted.

Substance Use and Gambling

The respondents report household use of betel nut (91), cigarettes (64), marijuana (4), alcohol (1) and heroin (2); most using daily. Of the 100 surveyed, 19 reported that substance use in self or family caused impediments in functioning. Gambling was reported in 11; all were husbands of women interviewed.

Work and Family Income

A total of 100 people represented by the survey worked for pay. Female adults and children tended to work as housekeepers, laborers or in garment piecework, while male adults and children tended to work as rickshaw pullers, laborers, brick breakers, drivers or carpenters. Male and female adults worked an average of 9 hours and 14 hours per day respectively, while male and female children work and average of 14 and 10 hours per day.

The families reported 35 of 228 children aged 6-18 worked for pay; 29 boys earned 1107 Taka per month and six girls earned 733 Taka per month. The average income per family was 3725 Taka per month and the average expenditure was 3218 per month, however 37 families reported expenses greater than income and dependence on loans for survival. Expenditures included rent, food, education, clothes, electricity, water, wood and health care.

DISCUSSION

This study describes the subsistence of 100 households, representing a total of 511 people living in the slums of Dhaka.

Subjects were largely migrants to Dhaka, living in small bamboo huts with an average of 3 children per household. They were uneducated, lived in unhygienic and difficult conditions worked in the informal service sector and consumed a diet low in protein. Health concerns included a variety of acute and chronic conditions both in the respondents and their children, and difficulties accessing health and dental care were reported.

The findings of this study are comparable to results of the 1995 Study of Urban Poverty in Bangladesh in which poverty was defined by monthly household income of 2264 BDT ($66 1995 USD) and 2313 households were evaluated. Compared to the present study, living conditions, prevalence of illness, access to clean water and latrines, availability of health services, nutrition, education, employment and security were similar or slightly better for the 1995 cohort. Other studies have also reported slum dwellers as comprising distressed migrants from rural areas, with poverty-driven Urbanisation due to unsustainable rural economy.

Consistent with a 1993 Unicef report, the main reasons for migration to Dhaka remain poverty, landlessness, unemployment and river erosion. The urban poor have been noted to pay very high rent for dismal housing, and dwellings in Dhaka are often on government-owned land; moving within slums is common due to land re-appropriation. Unsanitary latrine conditions are found in 76.6% and many pay intermediaries for utilities. As in other studies, pumped/tap water is used for drinking while open/surface water is used for non-drinking purposes. Childhood immunization in Dhaka slum households has been reported at 51-76%. In this survey 89% reported childhood immunization, though records for each child were not polled.

Adult access to immunizations was comparable to a study in the slum areas of Bangladesh, in which 85% had tetanus immunizations. Poor health literacy and maternal misperception of immunizations is common in Dhaka. Only 25% of mothers had received any formal education in one study. Half of the respondents in this study had a child die, an extremely high number, comparable to other samples of Dhaka slums, where 31-46% of mothers reported previous child death. In this as in other studies, symptoms rather than diagnoses of diseases were reported, and most causes of death were unknown in this study (39%) as in the literature (48%).

As in previous reports, most deaths occurred in the first year of life, and diarrhea was a frequent cause. Other causes in the literature and this study were respiratory illness and drowning. Neonatal tetanus was not a main cause of death here, perhaps due to immunization or symptom recognition. As in previous slum studies most sought treatment prior to their child's death. Lack of maternal education has previously been found to be a strong predictor of infant loss. A family member rather than a trained birth attendant assisted most births in the slums in this and other studies.

Only 5-10% of births are attended by someone trained in safe childbirth practices; even the most basic cleanliness is not observed, e.g. the umbilical cord is cut with an unsterilized razor or bamboo strip. In this study 47% of women delivered their babies in Dhaka, 51% in their village of origin and 2% in a hospital, compared to 69%, 28% and 3% in another study of births in Dhaka slums. At any given time, 30-45% of the urban poor have been reported ill. Barriers to care in the Dhaka slums have previously been noted to be accessibility, long distances to travel, a family's unwillingness to spend money on female care, providers prejudiced against the poor, short clinic hours, and cost. The poor may visit village doctors for convenience and low cost.

Family income per month in the Dhaka slums in USD has been reported at $71-82, $75 and $60 in past studies, comparable to the $63/month reported herein. Slum dwellers often work for wages much lower than those specified by law. Children in this study (12%) worked 10-14 hours/day and contributed to family income, similar to a 1993 Unicef report, where they were noted work an average of 10.7 hours/day. The BDHS is conducted every 4 years and is provides the most reliable national estimates of health, living conditions and conduct. It is data source for policymakers, programme managers, donors and researchers. Although urban areas are surveyed, slums are not specifically studied in any national survey even though half of Dhaka's population lives in the slums. Compared to BDHS data, household size was the same.

No education was recorded in one third of the BDHS, compared to 81% in our study. Homes were brick/cement in 54% compared to 2% herein, and 80% owned their homestead nationally compared to none of the slum dwellers. Electricity was in-home for 81.2%, compared to 34% in this survey. Toilets were sealed septic tanks for 65% of the BDHS population compared to none here, and over 50% in the BDHS reported adequate or surplus of food compared to 10% herein. Urban planning for health interventions and infrastructure for increasingly large slum areas will require study of this population as the BDHS tends to underestimate the severity of conditions.

There were considerable limitations of this pilot study, including the small study size, a tiny fraction of the 3.4 million in the slums of Dhaka. Slums are not uniform in their population or demographics, however the areas polled and results here are comparable to the Study of Urban Poverty in Bangladesh, as well as other studies of health and poverty in the Dhaka slums. As language and health literacy limit reliability, symptoms rather than diagnoses may better investigate these subjects. Few deaths are attended by physicians, however verbal autopsies have been found to be practical estimates. Finally, surveys are self-report, which leads to recall bias. Notably, the magnitude of memory lapse was not assessed, and immunization cards were not (in each case) documented by the surveyors.

AREAS OF FUTURE RESEARCH

By all counts, Urbanisation in Bangladesh is projected to increase, with an estimated 80 million living in urban areas by 2020, 40-60% of whom will be in the slums. This study and others show that these people are human capital greatly contributing to the economy and work force of the country. The majority migrated to Dhaka for economic reasons, and once there suffer unacceptable levels of malnutrition, hygiene and health, deprived of essential health services, financial stability, education and security. Bangladesh was slated as most corrupt in the 2002 Corruption Perceptions Index. Evidence in the slums is in payment by slum dwellers to land owners or managers for rent, utilities and security. This and ongoing costs for food and health services prevent economic advancement. Violence, coercion and extortion are part this system.

Slum living is an unavoidable reality of the future; efforts must be made to build the slums of Dhaka into sustainable communities. To accomplish this, a strategy involving government authorization to use the land and the creation of infrastructure and sustainable development with the elimination of corruption is crucial at all levels of government, police and individual slum leaders.

Essential service packages require focus for efficient service delivery. Incorporating NGOs into uniform healthcare and service delivery appears logical given that they already deliver three quarters of first contact care. Finally, numerous studies describe health and demographic data pointing to causes of poor health and livelihood in the Dhaka slums.

Conclusions generally identify the problem or risk factor and suggest that improvement of the variable in question will lead to improvements in outcomes e.g. improving nutrition is likely to reduce the incidence of diarrhea.

These problems though important are numerous, and it is unlikely that piecemeal solutions will be amply cost effective to achieve health in the slums; rather these problems require parallel attention. Funds are limited, and to alleviate poverty a detailed cost effectiveness analysis of comprehensive interventions is required, to create a strategy for sustainable improvements in the quality of life for those in the ever growing slums of Dhaka.

SLUMS DEMAND ACCESS TO CLEAN WATER

Kalyanpur - Rasheda Begum, a 25-year old garment factory worker, pays one Taka (58 Takas = US$1) and presses a hand pump to get a bucket of clean water from a water outlet, just around the corner from where she lives. One Taka for a 20-litre bucket of water is expensive considering that the municipality charges 4.50 Taka for 1,000 litres of water, but in this shantytown in Kalyanpur, a suburb of the Bangladesh capital Dhaka, it is a sign of progress for Mrs. Begum, who lives with her husband, small son and mother-in-law in a one-room tin shack.

Just five years ago the only sources of water for the slum's 500 families were wells and an intermittent supply from an illegally connected tap to the city's water utility. For drinking water, the women and children had to wait in line for up to two hours to collect a pitcher or bucket of water from a local market or nearby houses where they often had to bribe guards and caretakers, or pay exorbitant prices.

"We had to get up very early to get the water. We often incurred the wrath of husbands and in-laws when we were delayed," Mrs. Begum says.

Today the family uses water from a dug well behind their shack for bathing and washing, but for drinking and cooking, they get water from the slum's "water point"-two hand pumps that draw water from an underground reservoir that is filled with piped water supplied by Dhaka's water utility.

The shantytown, named No. 2 Pura Basti or Burned Slum after it was damaged in a fire 15 years ago, is a cluster of tin and bamboo shacks that line narrow cobbled lanes flanked by open gutters. The shacks have electricity, but no running water or gas supply. The women cook food over wood-fired earthen stoves outside their shacks. There are no proper sanitation facilities in the slum.

In PTC *Bast*, another city slum at Nakhalpara, an industrial zone in Dhaka, before the water point was installed, the women used to spend hours at night or early morning collecting water from nearby factories or housing estates. "We used to wait in line and sometimes suffer insults or beatings from the house owners," recalls Chan Banu.

The Begums are some of the three million people-or about a third-of Dhaka's 11 million people who live in slums. The working poor, who are most of the slum's inhabitants, earn their living as construction or factory workers, lorry drivers, rickshaw pullers, or work in informal sectors as domestic helps, or trash pickers.

Mrs. Begum earns 1,000 Takas month (about $17) making knitwear for export overseas, while her husband, Shah Alam, makes 1,800-2,100 Takas ($31-$36) monthly carrying passengers and goods in his three-wheel pedal rickshaw. Their eight-year-old son goes to a charity-financed school. The household's average monthly income is 3,000 Takas (about $52).

Most Bangladeshis live on less than a dollar a day. Every year, thousands of destitute victims of natural disasters pour into the cities from far-flung villages. The accelerated rate of Urbanisation means that nearly 25 percent of Bangladesh's 130 million people now live in urban areas, and municipalities and service agencies are unable to cope with the pressures of providing basic services.

Bangladesh has achieved remarkable success in supplying bacteria-free, safe drinking water to 97 percent of the population, mainly by sinking millions of shallow tube wells in the 1970s-80s. However, that success was undermined in the mid-1990s by the discovery of arsenic contamination of the groundwater, and it is estimated that 29 million of Bangladesh's 130 million people are still drinking arsenic-tainted water.

CLEAN WATER COMES TO THE SHANTYTOWN

Change came to the shantytown when a group of families got together and decided to ask a local nongovernmental organisation (NGO) for assistance in getting a proper and legal water connection. "We all suffered for lack of water five years ago. So we got together and took a decision," says Rabeya Akhter, a slum inhabitant.

The problem was that the Dhaka water agency was authorized only to provide services to legal landowners and residents and deemed slum-dwellers, who live illegally on public or private land, as non-existent clients. "We can only give water and sewerage connections to legal title holders of land or house owners," says Mohammad Nurul Huda Mian, commercial manager of the Dhaka water agency.

But the situation has changed, somewhat. Since it has been established that the people who live in slums are willing and able to pay, the water authority is no longer reluctant to give them a water connection. "The law doesn't permit it, but now the rules are relaxed a bit due to social considerations," says Mr. Mian.

The change has been accompanied, in large measure, by a 1988 national water policy that recognizes the right of transient people to receive water and sanitation services, and a change in the law is under active consideration. "We feel it is a basic human right to have water," says Mr. Mian. "We have to be practical. Slums will always be there and they need services. We must see slum inhabitants as potential clients who make a big contribution to society."

To work around the obstacles that prevented access to clean water, the residents of No. 2 Pura Basti approached a Dhaka-based NGO, *Dushtha Shasthya Kendra* (DSK) for help. DSK, an organisation that has been working to promote health, clean water supply and sanitation in poor areas of Dhaka since the late 1980s, has established 88 water points in 70 slums, benefiting more than 200,000 people. About a dozen water points have been paid for and handed over to the user groups.

"Slum dwellers are willing and able to pay for services, they are not asking for charity," says Masudul Quader, DSK's programme director. "Besides, free services don't work. If they pay, they feel more responsible for sustaining the services." In 1998, the United Nations Development Program (UNDP), through its Local Initiative Facility for Urban Environment or LIFE, joined forces with DSK to empower community-based organizations to make the projects sustainable. LIFE, which helps city dwellers help themselves by finding locally inspired solutions to local problems, funds small-scale, low-cost projects which are proposed, planned and executed by local communities.

"We help make communities more aware and strengthen their position to go ahead and demand more service provisions," says Tanzina Haque Hossain, national coordinator of LIFE in Bangladesh. LIFE in Bangladesh saw this work as an opportunity to popularize the idea of "local initiative." "The slum inhabitants contribute valuable services and capital to the city," says Ms. Hossain. "When they are empowered through information and organisation, you can see miracles happening-dirty lanes become clean, children get safe drinking water, and most of all, and people do not feel they are at the mercy of others all the time."

ESTABLISHING A WATER POINT

"When we visited the slum area to provide healthcare, they asked us for a water point," says Kalim Ullah, DSK's coordinator for water and sanitation projects. It took nearly a year of meetings with community members to assess their needs, select a site, fix rules for water use and rates, and outline management plans. But eventually, the slum had its water point approved by DSK.

To install the water point, DSK loaned the slum community nearly 43,000 Takas ($740), which was sponsored by an international donor agency. Thirty-four out of the slum's 500 families then formed a user group, which is charged with managing the water point and ensuring payment of water bills and loan installments to DSK. The user group annually elects a water-point operating committee consisting of nine women, who take care of the water point and collect payments.

The women members take turns each month to act as caretaker for the day-to-day running of the water point. In addition, a supporting advisory committee of five men is also elected annually to ensure security and maintenance of the water outlets, and to settle any disputes over bill payments. The 34-member families pay a fixed charge of 15 Takas per week for using the water, but they have learned not to overuse or waste. The committee also sells water to non-members, charging one Taka for a pitcher or bucket of water, and two Takas, for bathing or washing clothes.

The collection is used to repay the DSK loan, water bills, maintenance costs and the caretaker's honorarium. For the slum community, the piped water supply is still costly, yet it is far less than the two Takas, they had been paying for a 20-1itre pitcher or bucket. "Hopefully in another year, we will be able to pay off the loan. Then the water will be cheaper, even half the price," says Rabeya Akhter, who is the operating committee's current cashier.

According to DSK's Dibalok Singha, the water and sanitation improvements in the slums may not lead to long-term solutions, but they are still important. "Slums may be illegal and temporary. But we provide the inhabitants with a healthy standard of living, a better quality of life while they are still there."

SLUMS STILL WITHOUT SANITATION

About four years ago, the Dhaka city corporation, which owns the land, occupied by the No. 2 Pura Basti slam, paved the dirt lanes and installed some community toilets. But these basic latrines, which are concrete rings set in the ground without any water or flushing facilities, drain into an open gutter, which in turn is linked to a nearby pond. The area reeks of garbage and human waste.

The city did not assign anyone the responsibility of cleaning or maintaining the toilets. "There is no way to dispose of garbage or sewage that builds up behind the toilets, which are always blocked," says Rena Begum, a housewife with three children. "We have to close our eyes when inside, and have to get a bath afterward." Nearly 200-300 people, carrying pots of water, wait in long queues to use the toilets each morning, and bickering is common.

The children and the elderly, who cannot make it on time, defecate in the gutters outside their homes. "Before, we used makeshift latrines over the pond," says Mrs. Begum. Those latrines, she explained, were bamboo platforms hanging over the pond, curtained off by sackcloth for privacy. "Even that was better."

Bringing water to the shantytowns is one thing, using it properly is another? In an attempt to raise awareness of healthy practices, the LIFE programme supports visits by Shakila Akhter, a DSK community health worker, to No. 2 Pura Basti at least once a month. Using flash cards, she teaches proper use of water for cleaning, cooking and personal hygiene to members of the water point user group. At another meeting, Ms. Akhter reviews and evaluates the community's water sources and utilization, using posters and flow charts sketched on brown paper. "There are fewer outbreaks of diarrhoea and skin diseases, like scabies, in the slam now," Ms. Akhter reports.

Bibliography

Anne E. Beall and Robert J. Sternberg. *The Psychology of Gender*. New York: Gilford Press, 1993.

Anne Fausto-Sterling. *Myths of Gender: Biological Theories about Men and Women*. New York: Basic Books, 1985.

Bandura, Albert. *Social Learning Theory*. Englewood Cliffs, NJ:Prentice-Hall, 1977.

Beal, Carole R. *Boys and Girls: The Development of Gender Roles*. New York: McGraw-Hill, 1994.

Brett Beemyn and Mickey Eliason. *Queer Studies: A Lesbian, Gay, Bisexual, & Transgender Anthology*. New York: New York University Press, 1996.

Bridges, Judith S. "Pink or Blue: Gender-Stereotypic Perceptions of Infants as Conveyed by Birth Congratulations Cards." *Psychology of Women Quarterly* 17 (1993):193-205.

David D. Gilmore. *Manhood in the Making: Cultural Concepts of Masculinity*. New Haven, CT: Yale UP, 1990.

Denmark, Florence, Vita Rabinowitz, and Jeri Sechzer. *Engendering Psychology*. Boston: Allyn and Bacon, 2000.

Fagot, Beverly I., and Mary D. Leinbach. "The Young Child's Gender Schema: Environmental Input, Internal Organization." *Child Development* 60 (1989):663-672.

Felicity Haynes and Tarquam KcKenna. *Unseen Genders: Beyond the Binaries*. New York: 2001.

Gordene Olga MacKenzie. *Transgender Nation*. Bowling Green, OH: Bowling Green University Popular Press, 1994.

Halpern, Diane F. *Sex Differences in Cognitive Abilities*, 3rd edition. Mahwah, NJ: Lawrence Erlbaum, 2000.

Holly Devor. *Gender Blending: Confronting the Limits of Duality*. Bloomington, IN: Indiana UP, 1989.

John Money & Anke A. Ehrhardt. *Man & Woman, Boy & Girl*. Baltimore, MD: Johns Hopkins UP, 1972.

John Money & Patricia Tucker. *Sexual Signatures: On Being a Man or a Woman*. Boston, MA: Little, Brown, 1975.

John Stoltenberg. *The End of Manhood: A Book for Men of Conscience*. New York: Dutton, 1993.

Kohlberg, Lawrence. "A Cognitive-Developmental Analysis of Children's Sex Role Concepts and Attitudes." In Eleanor E. Maccoby ed., *The Development of Sex Differences*. Stanford, CA: Stanford University Press, 1966.

Letty Cottin Pogrebin. Growing Up Free: Raising Your Child in the 80's. New York: McGraw-Hill, 1980.

Maccoby, Eleanor E. *The Two Sexes: Growing Up Apart, Coming Together*. Cambridge, MA: Harvard University Press, Belknap Press, 1998.

Martin, Carol L., and Charles F. Halverson. "A Schematic Processing Model of Sex Typing and Stereotyping in Children." *Child Development* 52 (1981):1119-1134.

Pat Califia. *Public Sex: The Culture of Radical Sex*. San Francisco, CA: Cleis Press, 1994.

Pollack, William. *Real Boys*. New York: Henry Holt, 1998.

Rachel T. Hare-Mustin and Jeanne Marecek, eds. *Making a Difference: Psychology and the Construction of Gender*. New Haven, CT: Yale UP, 1990.

Rheingold, Harriet L., and Kaye V. Cook. "The Content of Boys' and Girls' Rooms as an Index of Parents' Behavior." *Child Development* 46 (1975):445-463.

Robert J. Stoller. *Sex and Gender: On the Development of Masculinity and Femininity*. New York: Science House, 1968.

Robert Moore and Douglas Gillette. *The King Within: Assessing the King in the Male Psyche*. New York: Morrow, 1992.

Sandra Lipsitz Bem. *The Lens of Gender: Transforming the Debate on Sexual Inequality*. New Haven, CT: Yale UP, 1993

Sandra Lipsitz Bem. *The Lens of Gender: Transforming the Debate on Sexual Inequality*. New Haven, CT: Yale UP, 1993.

Sherry B. Ortner and Harriet Whitehead, eds. *Sexual Meanings: The Cultural Construction of Gender and Sexuality*. Cambridge, UK: Cambridge UP, 1981.

Sherry B. Ortner and Harriet Whitehead. *Sexual Meanings: The Cultural Construction of Gender and Sexuality*. Cambridge, UK: Cambridge UP, 1981.

Stern, Marilyn, and Katherine H. Karraker. "Sex Stereotyping of Infants: A Review of Gender Labeling Studies." *Sex Roles* 20 (1989):501-522.

Susan Brownmiller. *Femininity*. New York: Linden Press/Simon & Schuster, 1984.

Susan Golombok & Robyn Fivush. *Gender Development*. Cambridge, UK: Cambridge UP, 1994.

Index